New Trends and Technologies in Facial Plastic Surgery

Editor

JASON D. BLOOM

FACIAL PLASTIC SURGERY CLINICS OF NORTH AMERICA

www.facialplastic.theclinics.com

Consulting Editor
J. REGAN THOMAS

August 2019 • Volume 27 • Number 3

ELSEVIER

1600 John F. Kennedy Boulevard • Suite 1800 • Philadelphia, Pennsylvania, 19103-2899

http://www.theclinics.com

FACIAL PLASTIC SURGERY CLINICS OF NORTH AMERICA Volume 27, Number 3
August 2019 ISSN 1064-7406, ISBN-13: 978-0-323-68238-1

Editor: Jessica McCool
Developmental Editor: Laura Kavanaugh

Facial Plastic Surgery Clinics of North America (ISSN 1064-7406) is published quarterly by Elsevier Inc., 360 Park Avenue South, New York, NY 10010-1710. Months of issue are February, May, August, and November. Business and Editorial Offices: 1600 John F. Kennedy Blvd., Suite 1800, Philadelphia, PA 19103-2899. Periodicals postage paid at New York, NY, and additional mailing offices. Subscription prices are $408.00 per year (US individuals), $659.00 per year (US institutions), $454.00 per year (Canadian individuals), $820.00 per year (Canadian institutions), $535.00 per year (foreign individuals), $820.00 per year (foreign institutions), $100.00 per year (US students), and $255.00 per year (foreign students). Foreign air speed delivery is included in all *Clinics* subscription prices. All prices are subject to change without notice. POSTMASTER: Send address changes to *Facial Plastic Surgery Clinics*, Elsevier Health Sciences Division, Subscription Customer Service, 3251 Riverport Lane, Maryland Heights, MO 63043. **Customer service: 1-800-654-2452 (US and Canada); 1-314-447-8871 (outside US and Canada); Fax: 314-447-8029; E-mail: journalscustomerservice-usa@elsevier.com (for print support); journalsonline support-usa@elsevier.com (for online support).**

Reprints. For copies of 100 or more of articles in this publication, please contact the Commercial Reprints Department, Elsevier Inc., 360 Park Avenue South, New York, NY 10010-1710. Tel.: 212-633-3874; Fax: 212-633-3820; E-mail: reprints@elsevier.com.

Facial Plastic Surgery Clinics of North America is covered in *MEDLINE/PubMed (Index Medicus)*.

Contributors

CONSULTING EDITOR

J. REGAN THOMAS, MD
Professor, Facial Plastic and Reconstructive
Surgery, Department of Otolaryngology–Head
and Neck Surgery, Northwestern University
Feinberg School of Medicine, Chicago, Illinois,
USA

EDITOR

JASON D. BLOOM, MD
Adjunct Assistant Professor, Department of
Otorhinolaryngology–Head and Neck Surgery,
Division of Facial Plastic Surgery, University of
Pennsylvania, Clinical Assistant Professor
(Adjunct), Department of Dermatology, Temple
University School of Medicine, Philadelphia,
Pennsylvania, USA; Director of Facial Plastic
and Reconstructive Surgery, Main Line Center
for Laser Surgery, Ardmore, Pennsylvania,
USA

AUTHORS

ASHLIN J. ALEXANDER, MD, FRCSC
Clinical Lecturer, Division of Facial Plastic and
Reconstructive Surgery, Department of
Otolaryngology–Head and Neck Surgery,
University of Toronto, Toronto, Ontario,
Canada

KAETE A. ARCHER, MD
Private Practice, Aesthetic Institute of
Manhattan for Facial and Plastic Surgery, New
York, New York, USA

ANTHONY BARED, MD, FACS
Private Practice, Miami, Florida, USA

CHRISTIAN H. BARNES, MD
Fellow, Facial Plastic and Reconstructive
Surgery, The Maas Clinic, San Francisco,
California, USA

ILAN BLOOM, BEng, MES
Douglas Hospital Research Center, McGill
University, Montreal, Quebec, Canada

JASON D. BLOOM, MD
Adjunct Assistant Professor, Department of
Otorhinolaryngology–Head and Neck Surgery,
Division of Facial Plastic Surgery, University of
Pennsylvania, Clinical Assistant Professor
(Adjunct), Department of Dermatology, Temple
University School of Medicine, Philadelphia,
Pennsylvania, USA; Director of Facial Plastic
and Reconstructive Surgery, Main Line Center
for Laser Surgery, Ardmore, Pennsylvania,
USA

ZACHARY FRIDIRICI, MD
Facial Plastic and Reconstructive Surgery
Fellow, Department of Otolaryngology–Head

and Neck Surgery, University of California, San Francisco, San Francisco, California, USA

ROBERTO ELOY GARCIA, MD, FACS
Private Practice, Contoura Facial Plastic Surgery, Ponte Vedra Beach, Florida, USA

RICHARD D. GENTILE, MD, MBA
Medical Director, Department of Facial Plastic Surgery, Gentile Facial Plastic Surgery and Aesthetic Laser Center, Youngstown, Ohio, USA; Staff Physician, Department of Facial Plastic Surgery, Cleveland Clinic Akron General Hospital, Akron, Ohio, USA

KIAN KARIMI, MD, FACS
Medical Director and Founder, Rejuva Medical Aesthetics, Los Angeles, California, USA

FRÉDÉRICK LALIBERTÉ, MD
Resident, Division of Facial Plastic and Reconstructive Surgery, Department of Otolaryngology–Head and Neck Surgery, University of Toronto, Toronto, Ontario, Canada

GARY LINKOV, MD
City Facial Plastics, New York, New York, USA

GARRETT D. LOCKETZ, MD
Department of Otolaryngology–Head and Neck Surgery, Division of Facial Plastic Surgery, University of Pennsylvania, Philadelphia, Pennsylvania, USA

COREY S. MAAS, MD
Facial Plastic and Reconstructive Surgery, The Maas Clinic, San Francisco, California, USA

UMANG MEHTA, MD
Mehta Plastic Surgery, Atherton, California, USA

SAM P. MOST, MD
Professor, Departments of Otolaryngology–Head and Neck Surgery and Surgery (Plastic Surgery), Director, Fellowship in Facial Plastic and Reconstructive Surgery, Chief, Division of Facial Plastic and Reconstructive Surgery, Stanford University School of Medicine, Stanford, California, USA

LAXMEESH MIKE NAYAK, MD
Nayak Plastic Surgery, St Louis, Missouri, USA

GRACE LEE PENG, MD, FACS
Facial Plastic and Reconstructive Surgery, Beverly Hills, California, USA

JORDAN RIHANI, MD, FACS
Facial Plastic Surgery Institute, Southlake, Texas, USA

HELENA ROCKWELL, BSc
Medical Assistant and Clinical Research Coordinator, Rejuva Medical Aesthetics, Los Angeles, California, USA

AKSHAY SANAN, MD
Clinical Instructor, Division of Facial Plastic and Reconstructive Surgery, Stanford University School of Medicine, Stanford, California, USA

SARMELA SUNDER, MD
Facial Plastic Surgeon, Beverly Hills, California, USA

BENJAMIN TALEI, MD, FACS
Director, Facial Plastic and Reconstructive Surgery, Beverly Hills Center for Plastic & Laser Surgery, Beverly Hills, California, USA

STEVEN F. WEINER, MD
Santa Rosa Beach, Florida, USA

Contents

Foreword: Emerging Trends, Techniques, and Technologies in Facial Plastic and Reconstructive Surgery   xi

J. Regan Thomas

Preface: Emerging Trends, Techniques, and Technologies in Facial Plastic and Reconstructive Surgery   xiii

Jason D. Bloom

Renuvion/J-Plasma for Subdermal Skin Tightening Facial Contouring and Skin Rejuvenation of the Face and Neck   273

Richard D. Gentile

The Renuvion/J-Plasma helium based plasma device from Apyx Medical has technological features that result in a unique and effective method of action for the contraction of subdermal soft tissue. The device achieves soft tissue contraction by instantly heating tissue to temperatures greater than 85°C for between 0.040 and 0.080 seconds. The tissue surrounding the treatment site remains at much cooler temperatures resulting in rapid cooling of the tissue through conductive heat transfer. Compared to bulk tissue heating devices, this method of action results in effective soft tissue contraction with a lower risk of injury to surrounding tissue.

Radiofrequency Microneedling: Overview of Technology, Advantages, Differences in Devices, Studies, and Indications   291

Steven F. Weiner

Radiofrequency (RF) skin rejuvenation is improved using RF microneedling (RFM) devices. More aggressive treatments are performed safely with minimal downtime than previous RF devices. Optimizing treatment parameters is essential for safety and efficacy. Multiple RFM studies support minimal risks even in dark skin types. RFM has been used to treat acne scarring successfully as well as skin laxity and hyperhidrosis.

Percutaneous Radiofrequency Technologies for the Lower Face and Neck   305

Garrett D. Locketz and Jason D. Bloom

 Video content accompanies this article at http://www.facialplastic.theclinics.com.

The aging neck is one of the most common motivations for patients to seek aesthetic rejuvenation. Increasingly, patients are desiring less invasive aesthetic treatments with less morbidity and downtime. Percutaneous radiofrequency technologies have been recently introduced for cervical rejuvenation. These technologies safely and effectively apply energy directly into the subdermal space, targeting the upper dermal collagen network, the deeper fascial layer, and the fibrofatty septum that anchors the dermis to the deep fascia. Significant skin tightening and fat reduction have been reported with these technologies, beyond that which is currently achievable with other minimally invasive energy-based technologies.

Microfat and Nanofat: When and Where These Treatments Work   321

Jordan Rihani

Facial fat transfer has evolved from simple grafting techniques to smaller lobule (microfat) and adipose-derived stem cell (nanofat) injection techniques. These new methods look to overcome the early limitations of facial fat transfer while meeting increased demand and understanding of the role of volume loss in facial aging. The purpose of this article is to review basic principles of microfat and nanofat and demonstrate one technique for their application.

The Benefits of Platelet-Rich Fibrin   331

Kian Karimi and Helena Rockwell

 Video content accompanies this article at http://www.facialplastic.theclinics.com.

Platelet-rich fibrin (PRF) is a next-generation autologous platelet therapy with immense potential in several medical fields. In cosmetic medicine, for example, PRF is useful in wound healing and skin rejuvenation as a primary and a supplemental technique owing to its fibrin matrix, cellular components, and prolonged release of growth factors. PRF is simple to obtain, inexpensive, and may be administered topically, injected, or in conjunction with other esthetic procedures. In this regard, PRF possesses diverse, and increasingly pertinent capacities in esthetic medicine and surgery.

Silhouette Instalift: Benefits to a Facial Plastic Surgery Practice   341

Kaete A. Archer and Roberto Eloy Garcia

Absorbable suture suspension is one of the newest minimally invasive treatment trends for lifting and repositioning ptotic facial tissue. The Silhouette Instalift is a convenient in-office procedure that provides a unique and advanced clinical treatment for a natural looking midfacial lift. Research has shown that most patients characterized the Silhouette Instalift as immediately effective and were pleased by enhancements. The procedure has an improved safety and efficacy profile over the predecessor, barbed suture thread lifting, coupled with reduced risk of complications and recovery time compared with rhytidectomy. Absorbable suture suspension should be considered a workhorse in nonsurgical esthetic treatments.

Advanced Techniques in Nonsurgical Rhinoplasty   355

Umang Mehta and Zachary Fridirici

 Video content accompanies this article at http://www.facialplastic.theclinics.com.

For a multitude of reasons, facial plastic surgeons should be adept and comfortable with nonsurgical rhinoplasty. An intimate knowledge of nasal vascular anatomy, filler choice, and proper placement can make this a safe, effective, and long-lasting treatment. Basic techniques include dorsal augmentation and camouflaging of a dorsal hump. Advanced maneuvers are also possible, including increasing tip rotation and projection, straightening the nose, lowering alar rims, and potentially the improvement of nasal function.

A Bioabsorbable Lateral Nasal Wall Stent for Dynamic Nasal Valve Collapse: A Review   367

Akshay Sanan and Sam P. Most

Nasal obstruction is one of the most common clinical problems encountered by otolaryngologists and facial plastic surgeons. Lateral wall insufficiency (LWI) is a key anatomic contributor to nasal obstruction. Traditional techniques for correcting LWI include alar batten grafts, bone-anchored sutures, and lateral crural strut grafts. Latera is an absorbable nasal implant that can be inserted in the office or the operating room as an adjunctive procedure for LWI. The purpose of this review is to discuss Latera, a novel bioabsorbable implant to improve the nasal airway.

Social Media Marketing in Facial Plastic Surgery: What Has Worked?   373

Laxmeesh Mike Nayak and Gary Linkov

Social media is becoming one of the main avenues for direct consumer marketing. Patients use social media to find surgeons and to communicate about procedures, outcomes, and their experiences. A surgeon's social media presence can dramatically increase their perception of being an expert and showcase to patients their style and approach. There is no single best social network, instead various networks exist with unique characteristics that each have the potential to drive traffic to a practice. Social media can be potentially hazardous for patients and surgeons if misused.

What's New in Facial Hair Transplantation?: Effective Techniques for Beard and Eyebrow Transplantation   379

Anthony Bared

Natural results in facial hair restoration are made possible with modern refinements in hair transplantation. There has been a large increase in the demand for facial hair restoration in men and women. Women mostly seek to thicken and restore eyebrow density, whereas men seek to have a fuller beard. This article describes the techniques refined in facial hair transplantation.

The Modified Upper Lip Lift: Advanced Approach with Deep-Plane Release and Secure Suspension: 823-Patient Series   385

Benjamin Talei

The modified upper lip lift procedure is a simple evolution of the cutaneous bullhorn subnasal lip lift. The superficial muscular aponeurotic system layer in the lip is described along with the pyriform ligament, both of which play an essential role in lip lifting. This article details an easily reproducible deep-plane technique that can be applied to patients of all ages, ethnicities, and skin types.

The Critical Role of Nutrition in Facial Plastic Surgery   399

Frédérick Laliberté, Ilan Bloom, and Ashlin J. Alexander

Nutrition plays a key role in optimizing healing following surgery. The increased catabolic state postoperatively, coupled with a propensity for patients to be suffering from marginal nutritional deficiencies at baseline preoperatively, necessitates that the surgeon be attuned to the need for optimal perioperative nutritional support.

This ensures the smoothest recovery and best possible outcomes in facial plastic surgery. Key nutrients include vitamin A, vitamin C, zinc, bromelain, arnica montana, arginine, glutamine, hydrolyzed collagen, vitamin B complex, and protein. The ability for patients to obtain this optimal supplementation in a single product is the ideal solution for both surgeon and patient.

Platelet-Rich Plasma for Skin Rejuvenation: Facts, Fiction, and Pearls for Practice

405

Grace Lee Peng

Platelet-rich plasma (PRP) has gained popularity in facial plastic surgery because of its role in wound healing. PRP, having a higher concentration of platelets, allows for greater release of growth factors and biologically active proteins, which in turn activates the wound-healing cascade stimulating neoangiogenesis and collagen production. One of the most popular uses for PRP is for facial skin rejuvenation in the form of dermal injections and topical application during microneedling. The promising nature of PRP makes using it for injection and/or in conjunction with microneedling a good addition to any practice that deals with skin rejuvenation.

Relevant Topical Skin Care Products for Prevention and Treatment of Aging Skin

413

Sarmela Sunder

Options for skin care are varied. New products are introduced constantly and it is important for the practitioner to have an understanding of products that impart beneficial results for aging skin. Educating patients to use products with scientifically proven benefits leads to better outcomes. Patients should be encouraged to use daily sunscreen, a topical retinoid every night, and a topical antioxidant daily. Supplementing the routine skin care regimen with alpha hydroxy acids, growth factors, heparin sulfate, and defensins can be addressed individually. Exogenous stem cells do not have sufficient evidence to warrant recommending them currently.

Autologous Fat Harvest and Preparation for Optimal Predictable Outcomes

419

Christian H. Barnes and Corey S. Maas

 Video content accompanies this article at http://www.facialplastic.theclinics.com.

Best practices in fat transfer to the face focus on tissue harvest and processing techniques. This article discusses the role of adipose-derived mesenchymal stem cells (MSCs) in mitigating tissue loss in grafting. Discrepancies among common practice and recent study results have propagated uncertainty with long-term results. Fortunately, recent increases in the understanding of these MSCs are leading providers to identify statistically more favorable tissue donor sites, harvest technique, and preparation methods to increase their concentration in transferred tissue. Future studies are needed to support or confound the long-term effects of MSC transfer on facial fat grafting.

FACIAL PLASTIC SURGERY CLINICS OF NORTH AMERICA

FORTHCOMING ISSUES

November 2019
Revision Facial Plastic Surgery: Correcting Bad Results
Paul S. Nassif and Julia L. Kerolus, *Editors*

February 2020
Update of Today's Facial Skin Rejuvenation Technology
Richard D. Gentile, *Editor*

May 2020
Techniques for Hair Restoration
Lisa E. Ishii and Linda Lee, *Editors*

RECENT ISSUES

May 2019
Facial Gender Affirmation Surgery
Michael T. Somenenk, *Editor*

February 2019
Skin Cancer Treatment
Jeffrey S. Moyer, *Editor*

November 2018
Current Utilization of Biologicals
Gregory S. Keller, *Editor*

SERIES OF RELATED INTEREST

Clinics in Plastic Surgery
https://www.plasticsurgery.theclinics.com/
Otolaryngologic Clinics
https://www.oto.theclinics.com/

THE CLINICS ARE AVAILABLE ONLINE!
Access your subscription at:
www.theclinics.com

Foreword
Emerging Trends, Techniques, and Technologies in Facial Plastic and Reconstructive Surgery

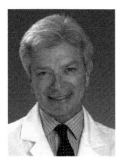

J. Regan Thomas, MD
Consulting Editor

Our specialty of Facial Plastic and Reconstructive Surgery is in a period of active and innovative change in technology as well as in techniques. The *Facial Plastic Surgery Clinics of North America* is pleased to present to our readership this issue, which focuses on those changes as presented by our guest editor, Jason Bloom, MD, and his contributing authors.

The authors demonstrate both surgical and nonsurgical procedures that are becoming increasingly useful and common in practice. Included are a variety of lasers and other energy-based treatment modalities, which are increasingly popular. The reader will potentially be introduced to new procedures to add to their practices as well as to compare procedures that they are utilizing with other experienced practitioners' approaches.

This issue of *Facial Plastic Surgery Clinics of North America* is part of the ongoing process to maintain an up-to-date and insightful, experienced understanding of key components utilized in the practice of modern facial plastic surgery. I am confident that this issue will fulfill those goals for our readers.

J. Regan Thomas, MD
Facial Plastic and Reconstructive Surgery
Department of Otolaryngology
Head and Neck Surgery
Northwestern University School of Medicine
675 North Saint Clair Street
Suite 15-200
Chicago, IL 60611, USA

E-mail address:
jreganthomas@gmail.com

Facial Plast Surg Clin N Am 27 (2019) xi
https://doi.org/10.1016/j.fsc.2019.04.011
1064-7406/19/© 2019 Published by Elsevier Inc.

Preface

Emerging Trends, Techniques, and Technologies in Facial Plastic and Reconstructive Surgery

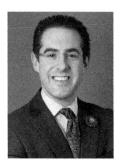

Jason D. Bloom, MD
Editor

This is a very exciting time for facial plastic surgery and aesthetic and cosmetic medicine. The market as a whole continues to grow by leaps and bounds each year, and facial plastic surgeons are at the forefront of innovation, clinical practice, and research with respect to the industry's growth. It is increasingly important for facial plastic surgeons to continue to stay informed of the research and clinical efforts that are taking place in this field because novel technologies and innovations are fueling advances in the profession.

The goal of this issue of *Facial Plastic Surgery Clinics of North America* is to provide information about cutting-edge ideas and techniques that some of the leaders in our specialty have already incorporated into their own practices. This will allow those who read this issue to make informed decisions about whether to adopt these new technologies and/or techniques in their own offices.

A portion of this issue is devoted to new energy-based technology and devices. With respect to these lasers and energy-based devices, technology is also moving at a rapid pace. At this time,

we are seeing minimally invasive devices that are helping to achieve excellent results with less downtime than previously seen. For example, one of these technologies includes combining radiofrequency microneedling systems and percutaneous energy-based devices to tighten down neck and jowl soft tissue. The results from some of these procedures are outstanding, and the results would never have been possible without surgery just a few years ago.

Another portion of this issue is devoted to new and innovative surgical and nonsurgical procedures and techniques that are gaining popularity more than ever before, including techniques that reduce surgical complications and improve outcomes. For example, this issue discusses a new implantable device designed to help patients breathe better, the latest in facial hair restoration, and nonsurgical treatments that enable a patient to "try out" a rhinoplasty before opting for surgery.

Finally, trends in facial plastic surgery and the aesthetic industry are constantly changing. New

Facial Plast Surg Clin N Am 27 (2019) xiii–xiv
https://doi.org/10.1016/j.fsc.2019.04.010

marketing trends are utilized to attract new patients to practices and/or to market to existing patients. Other novel ideas include nonsurgical adjuncts like surgical nutrition options and post-surgery healing methods, which help patients reduce their downtime, improve their skin health, and optimize their overall results. These are implemented into practices to improve patient care, reduce adverse events, and make it easier to deliver treatments.

I am hopeful that this issue will provide thoughtful commentary about some of the innovations and advances that are currently happening in our industry. While it can be interesting to experiment with new techniques and technology, we as doctors, must weigh the positives and negatives of each of these options for our own practices. Our ultimate goal should be to associate with things that help our offices run smoother and to show significant clinical efficacy and improved results with minimal morbidity for our patients.

Jason D. Bloom, MD
Department of Otorhinolaryngology
Head and Neck Surgery
University of Pennsylvania
Philadelphia, PA 19104, USA

Department of Dermatology
Temple University School of Medicine
Philadelphia, PA 19140, USA

Main Line Center for Laser Surgery
32 Parking Plaza
Suite 200
Ardmore, PA 19003, USA

E-mail address:
drjbloom@hotmail.com

Renuvion/J-Plasma for Subdermal Skin Tightening Facial Contouring and Skin Rejuvenation of the Face and Neck

Richard D. Gentile, MD, MBA[a,b,*]

KEYWORDS

- Renuvion • J-plasma • Helium • Plasma • Subdermal • Coagulation • Collagen contraction
- Skin tightening

KEY POINTS

- Renuvion/J-Plasma offers unique benefits compared with CO_2 laser and conventional electrosurgical devices.
- Renuvion key benefits include low risk of injury to surrounding tissue.
- The Renuvion retractable blade enables greater versatility and control of the energy as well as enhanced visibility at the application site. Pistol-grip and pencil hand pieces with single-button cutting, dissection, ablation, and coagulation.

INTRODUCTION

Energy has been applied in some form to tissue since the beginning of recorded history. The practice of applying heat to tissue with the use of cautery was used for thousands of years as an invaluable method of controlling hemorrhage. Continuous improvement of methods for using the beneficial effects of heat on tissue eventually led to the development of the basic concepts of electrosurgery known today. In October 1926, Dr Harvey Cushing used an electrosurgical unit developed by Dr William T. Bovie to successfully remove a highly vascularized brain tumor from a patient after previous failed attempts. Today, electrosurgical instruments are used in almost every surgical procedure performed worldwide.[1] Skin tightening occurs because of the wound-healing cascade that occurs with tissue injury whether the wounding occurs by surgical, thermal, or chemical trauma. The end of collagen contraction and skin tightening occurs in the last phase of wound healing as realignment of collagen bundles permits overall contraction of the soft tissue and skin mass to occur. In this article, the authors examine the ability of a new class of cold atmospheric plasma (CAP) devices named Renuvion/JPlasma to improve skin tightening of facial, nasal, and cervical skin, including rhinophyma, and discuss and evaluate the technology's ability to offer neck and jowl sculpting and contouring in a manner that is both efficacious and safe. The authors also introduce evidence for potential

Disclosure Statement: Funding for animal studies was from Apyx Medical.
[a] Department of Facial Plastic Surgery, Gentile Facial Plastic Surgery & Aesthetic Laser Center, 821 Kentwood Suite C, Youngstown, OH 44512, USA; [b] Department of Facial Plastic Surgery, Cleveland Clinic Akron General Hospital, Akron, OH, USA
* Corresponding author. Department of Facial Plastic Surgery, Gentile Facial Plastic Surgery & Aesthetic Laser Center, 821 Kentwood Suite C, Youngstown, OH 44512.
E-mail address: dr-gentile@msn.com

applications for the treatment of cutaneous malignancies.

HISTORICAL BACKGROUND OF PLASMA TECHNOLOGIES IN MEDICINE AND SURGERY

Historically, plasmas were first used in a "biological" application in the late 1850s when Siemens used a dielectric-barrier discharge to generate ozone and used the ozone to clean water from biological contaminants. No systematic research was conducted to understand the interaction between plasmas and biological cells until more than 130 years later, in the mid-1990s. The credit of first description of plasma is attributed to William Crookes, who identified plasma in 1879. Of the visible universe, 99% is made up of plasma, referred to as the fourth state of matter (Fig. 1). The other states of matter are liquid, gas, and solid. In 1929, Dr Irvine Langmuir was the first to apply the word "plasma" to ionized gas. In the meantime, some attempts were made to use plasmas for biological sterilization from the 1960s to the 1980s.[2–4] Most of these experiments used plasma as a secondary agent in the sterilization process, and no scientific investigations were made to understand how plasma interacted with bacterial cells and how it caused their demise. In the early 1990s, a group at Los Alamos National Laboratory studied laser-produced plasmas for medical applications, including in ophthalmology, urology, and cardiology.[5] Because this new research topic of biomedical applications of plasmas was at its infancy in the early and mid-1990s, particularly in the case of atmospheric plasmas, not many people in the scientific community were aware of this work and funding was practically nonexistent. This initial funding was provided by the Electronics and Physics Directorate of the US Air Force Office of Scientific Research under a small business technology transfer program directed by Dr Robert J. Barker. In 1998, the International Conference on Plasma Science was held as the first session dedicated to disseminating the first results of a coordinated effort to investigate plasma-cell interactions.[6] In a few years' time, all major international plasma

Changes in States of Matter

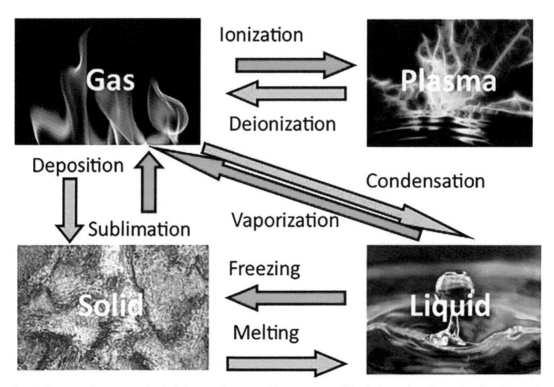

Fig. 1. Changes of state are physical changes in matter. They are reversible changes that do not involve changes in matter's chemical makeup or chemical properties.

conferences followed suit. Today, research has expanded to include work on the interaction of plasma with eukaryotic cells, such as mammalian cells, with potential applications in wound healing and in fighting some types of cancers by inducing apoptosis (programmed cell death). Renuvion are exciting applications that could take plasmas further into the medical and therapeutic fields and added the biological/medical applications of plasmas to their technical topics' repertoire.

COLD HELIUM (ATMOSPHERIC) PLASMAS APPLICATIONS AND DEVICE DEVELOPMENT

There are 2 types of plasma: thermal and nonthermal or CAP. Thermal plasma has electrons and heavy particles (neutrons and ions) at the same temperature. CAP is said to be nonthermal because it has electrons at a hotter temperature than the heavy particles that are at room temperature. In the usual description, the terms CAP and cold helium plasma (CHP) represent the same entity if helium gas is used for the generation of the CAP. For this purpose, CAP and CHP will be used synonymously to describe the use of helium-generated CAP. There are several methods to produce CAP, such as dielectric barrier discharge, , plasma needle, and plasma pencil. Several different gases can be used to produce CAP, such as helium, argon, nitrogen, heliox (a mix of helium and oxygen), and air. Because of the ability of CAP to deactivate microorganisms, cause cell detachment, and cause death in cancer cells, the earliest research on CAP has been in finding uses for CAP in dentistry and oncology. Koinuma and colleagues[7] developed the earliest radiofrequency (RF) cold plasma jet in 1992. The cathode is a needle electrode made of tungsten or stainless steel with a 1-mm diameter connected to an RF source (13.56 MHz). The needle electrode lies within a quartz tube, whereas the anode electrode is grounded. Depending on the application, helium or argon was mixed with various gases. This group published several articles describing its variants and applications of the plasma jet.[8–16] In 2002, Stoffels and colleagues[15] created a miniature atmospheric plasma jet that they called plasma needle and created a new version in 2004.[16] In the former version, the needle was enclosed in a box, and as a result, the samples had to be placed inside of the box to be treated. In the new version, the plasma needle consists of a 0.3-mm metal strand diameter with a sharpened tip inside of a Perspex tube. The length of the entire needle is 8 cm, and 1.5 cm remains uncovered by the Perspex tube. The gas used most frequently is helium because of its high thermal conductivity. The gas is then mixed with air at the needle tip, where a micro-discharge is created. Gases other than helium are also used.[17] The diameter of the plasma glow generated is 2 mm. Microplasma is created when RF power at 13.05 MHz ranging between 10 mW and several watts is applied to the needle. Its small size enables it to be used to treat small areas where accuracy is required. The microplasma device used for the patients reported in this article is produced by Bovie Medical Corporation (BMC) and is known as Renuvion/J-Plasma. In 1998, the BMC research team attended a conference in Dusseldorf, Germany, where it came across a plasma-based technology developed in Russia that appeared promising. BMC entered into a joint venture agreement to develop and bring the product to market. In 2007, BMC bought out its partner and continued development on its own. That product became Renuvion/J-Plasma, which uses a gas ionization process to produce a stable, focused beam of ionized gas that provides surgeons with greater precision, minimal invasiveness, and an absence of conductive currents during surgery. Once BMC took the development of J-Plasma in house, the device began coming together. In 2010, the team added J-Plasma's retractable blade, which allows it to function as a cutting tool that leaves behind almost no tissue damage. By early 2012, J-Plasma had received 510K Food and Drug Administration (FDA) clearance for cutting, coagulating, and ablating soft tissue. In aesthetics, the most recognized plasma device in recent history was the Rhytec Portrait PSR3 released in 2006, which is a resurfacing device only and does not permit cutting. The Portrait device is nitrogen based and is more highly ionized in the process than helium plasma, thus affecting the temperature. RF energy converts nitrogen gas into plasma within the hand piece. Rapid heating of the skin occurs as the plasma rapidly gives up energy to the skin. This energy transfer is not chromophore dependent. Another aesthetic device used by the senior author and offered in the early 2000s was Arthrocare Corporations' Visage, which used saline as the medium for plasma generation. Visage was used primarily for skin rejuvenation.

RENUVION/J-PLASMA OXIDATIVE STRESS AND ASSOCIATED BIOCHEMICAL CONSIDERATIONS

CAP is a highly reactive (partially) ionized physical state containing a mixture of physical and biologically active agents and varying degrees of thermal energy. Cold plasma generates radical species by the interaction of the plasma beam (H) with the surrounding air (N_2, O_2) or the water in the tissue (H_2O). The radical species are formed by cold plasma interaction by breaking apart 1 molecule and combining it into a new fragment, as they steal electrons from other molecules. New fragments provide some very unique effects. The most important components for biological effects include singlet oxygen ($^1O_2$), superoxide (O_2^-), ozone (O_3), hydroxyl radicals ($^\bullet OH$), useful in programmed cell death (apoptosis), nitrogen radicals ($N_2^\bullet$), nitric oxide ($^\bullet NO$), a powerful signaling molecule in inflammation and cellular injury response, nitrogen dioxide ($^\bullet NO_2$), peroxynitrite ($ONOO^-$), hydrogen peroxide (H_2O_2), also useful in apoptosis, organic radicals, electrons, energetic ions, and charged particles ($RO^\bullet$, $RO_2^\bullet$).[18] It is well known that reactive oxygen species (ROS) and reactive nitrogen species (RNS) can induce cell proliferation as well as cell death, while extreme amounts of reactive oxygen and nitrogen species can induce apoptosis and damage of proteins, lipids, and DNA. These interactions can induce epigenetic modifications at the cellular level. Oxidative stress, also known as the intracellular redox balance, is the disequilibrium between the ROS and RNS and the antioxidants, caused by a natural physiologic process in the biological system, where the presence of these free radicals overpowers the scavenging mechanisms. The uncontrolled production of ROS will eventually interact with molecular structures, such as DNA, proteins, lipids, and carbohydrates, leading to an alteration of the metabolic pathway activity. This effect will cause molecular damage, which will eventually result in the pathogenesis of different diseases, such as cancer, neurodegenerative diseases, and diabetes, as well as aging. Cancer cells are more susceptible to oxidative stress than healthy cells. CAP shows its promising potential to be a selective anticancer tool. Preliminary research over the past decade demonstrated that CAP could effectively inhibit the growth of dozens of cancer cell lines in vitro by mainly triggering apoptosis.[19] CAP is also capable of effectively resisting the growth of subcutaneously implanted xenograft tumors in mice by an unknown mechanism. The CAP-originated reactive species has been regarded as the primary factors resulting in cell death, although physical factors of CAP may also have minor unknown functions. Despite the fact that the anticancer molecular mechanism is still far from clear, current studies reveal that the apoptosis of CAP-treated cancer cells in vitro is mainly due to the intense DNA double-strand break caused by a significant increase of intracellular ROS. The differential expression of the aquaporin channels and intracellular antioxidant enzymes such as catalases in cancer cells and normal cells may be a plausible mechanism to control the selective diffusion of reactive species across the cytoplasmic membrane of cancer cells and selective increase of intracellular ROS in cancer cells. Because corresponding homologous normal cells just experience a weak increase of ROS, CAP can selectively cause apoptosis in cancer cells in vitro. Cold plasma is currently being studied for the antineoplastic properties and may be useful in treating cutaneous malignancies (**Fig. 2**).

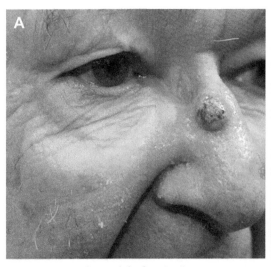 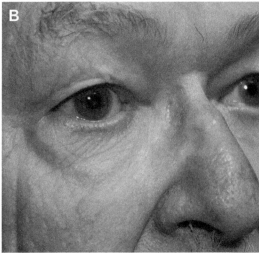

Fig. 2. Patient with a nodular basal cell carcinoma successfully treated with CAP/J-Plasma. (*A*) Nodular BCC (*B*) Post Excision nodular BCC. (*Courtesy of* J. B. Delozier III, MD, FACS, Nashville, TN.)

RENUVION DEVICE OVERVIEW AND SETTINGS

Renuvion/J-Plasma from the BMC represents a new approach to electrosurgery, whereby helium gas plasma, fueled by electrosurgical energy, flows into the application site for only a brief interval and then disperses out, leaving very precise, predictable effects. There is no net flow of electricity around the body, so no return electrode is required. The cold plasma effect is highly localized, minimizing collateral damage to surrounding healthy tissue (**Fig. 3**). Renuvion, having no need for a grounding pad, differentiates Renuvion from standard electrosurgical devices. Renuvion uses nonconductive currents and limits direct injury with its reduced tissue spread, minimizing the risk of direct and capacitive coupling. The Renuvion retractable blade (**Fig. 4**) enables greater versatility and control of the energy as well as enhanced visibility at the energy application on site. In addition, Renuvion allows for safe and effective tissue coagulation/ablation/incision with controlled precision when ablating tissue and reduced fear of injury to surrounding healthy structures. The thermal ablation zones of Renuvion are demonstrated in **Fig. 3** and compared with standard current-based electrosurgical ablation zones.

The Renuvion helium device has minimal lateral and depth of thermal spread in a variety of tissue types and comparisons with different devices and is shown graphically and histologically (**Figs. 5** and **6**). A comparison of the ablation zones in peritoneum is shown comparing Renuvion with conventional electrosurgical devices (**Fig. 7**). The thermal dispersion of the device increases linearly with increased power setting, gas flow rate, and exposure time in various tissue types. The depth of tissue effect with Renuvion ranges from no visible effect to about 2.0 mm with lateral spread ranging between 1.0 mm and 4.0 mm total diameter with typical use.[20]

Renuvion/J-Plasma Subdermal Method of Action

Through this long history, the heat effects of the RF alternating current used in electrosurgery on cells and tissue have been well established. Normal body temperature is 37°C and, with normal illness, can increase to 40°C without permanent impact or damage to the cells of the body. However, when the temperature of cells in tissue reaches 50°C, cell death occurs in approximately 6 minutes.[21] When the temperature of cells in tissue reaches 60°C, cell death occurs

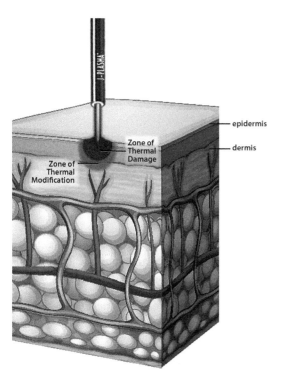

Fig. 3. Precise thermal ablation zones demonstrated with CAP/J-Plasma. (*Courtesy of* Apyx Medical, Clearwater, FL.)

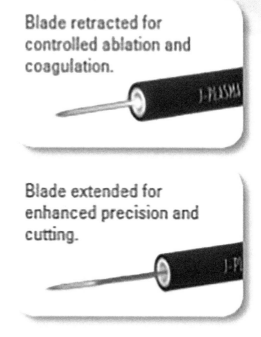

Blade retracted for controlled ablation and coagulation.

Blade extended for enhanced precision and cutting.

Fig. 4. There are different device configurations for the CAP/J-Plasma device, but all are equipped with a retractable blade or needle for tissue interface. (*Courtesy of* Apyx Medical, Clearwater, FL.)

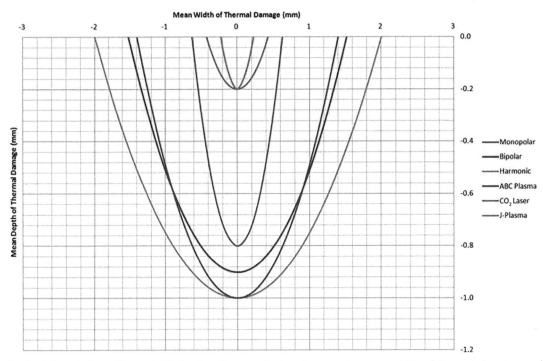

Fig. 5. Adjacent tissue thermal effects of various surgical devices. x-axis, mean width of thermal damage; and y-axis, mean depth of thermal damage. (*Data from* Bovie Medical Corporation, 2014.)

instantaneously.[22] Between the temperatures of 60°C and just below 100°C, 2 simultaneous processes occur.[1] The first is protein denaturation leading to coagulation, which is discussed in more detail later. The second is desiccation or dehydration, because the cells lose water through the thermally damaged cellular wall. As temperatures increase above 100°C, intracellular water turns to steam, and tissue cells begin to vaporize because of the massive intracellular expansion that occurs. Finally, at temperatures of 200°C or more, organic molecules are broken down into a process called carbonization. This carbonization leaves behind carbon molecules that give a black and/or brown appearance to the tissue. Understanding these heat effects of RF energy on cells and tissue can allow the predictable changes to be used to accomplish beneficial therapeutic results. Protein denaturation leading to soft tissue coagulation is one of the most versatile and widely used tissue effects. Protein denaturation is the process in which hydrothermal bonds (crosslinks) between protein molecules, such as collagen, are instantaneously broken and then quickly reformed as tissue cools. This process leads to the formation of uniform clumps of

protein typically called coagulum through a subsequent process known as coagulation. In the process of coagulation, cellular proteins are altered but not destroyed and form protein bonds that create homogenous, gelatinous structures. The resulting tissue effect of coagulation is extremely useful and most commonly used for occluding blood vessels and causing hemostasis. In addition to causing hemostasis, coagulation results in predictable contraction of soft tissue. Collagen is one of the main proteins found in human skin and connective tissue. The coagulation/denaturation temperature of collagen is conventionally stated to be 66.8°C, although this can vary for different tissue types.[23] Once denatured, collagen rapidly contracts as fibers shrink to one-third of their overall length.[24] However, the amount of contraction depends on the temperature and the duration of the treatment. The hotter the temperature, the shorter the amount of treatment time needed for maximal contraction.[25] For example, collagen heated at a temperature of 65°C must be heated for greater than 120 seconds for significant contraction to occur, but at a temperature of 85°C, maximal contraction occurs in approximately 0.044 seconds.[25]

Peritoneum

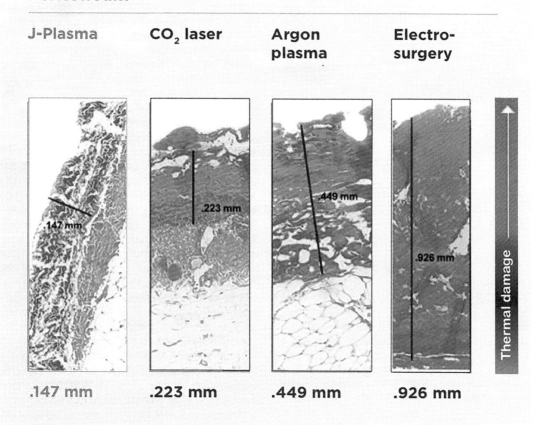

J-Plasma	CO$_2$ laser	Argon plasma	Electro-surgery
.147 mm	.223 mm	.449 mm	.926 mm

Fig. 6. A tissue sample of devices and adjacent thermal damage. (H&E stains at 100×).

This principle of thermally induced contraction of collagen through denaturation and coagulation of soft tissue is well known in medicine and is used to achieve beneficial results in ophthalmology, orthopedic applications, the treatment of varicose veins, and cosmetic plastic surgery procedures. Once tissue is heated to the appropriate temperature, protein denaturation and collagen contraction occur, resulting in a reduction of volume and surface area of the heated tissue. Noninvasive use of RF devices, lasers, and plasma devices has been used for the reduction of facial wrinkles and rhytids caused by thermal-induced collagen/tissue contraction since the mid-1990s.[26–31]

Recently, the use of thermal-induced collagen/tissue contraction has been expanded to minimally invasive procedures. Laser-assisted lipolysis and radiofrequency-assisted lipolysis (RFAL) devices have combined the removal of subcutaneous fat with soft tissue heating to reduce the skin laxity that often results from fat volume removal. These devices are placed in the same subcutaneous tissue plane as a standard suction-assisted lipolysis cannula and are used to deliver thermal energy to coagulate the subcutaneous tissue, including the underside of the dermis, the fascia, and the septal connective tissue. The coagulation of the subcutaneous tissue results in collagen/tissue contraction that reduces skin laxity. BMC's Renuvion (formerly branded as J-Plasma) helium-based plasma technology has FDA clearance for the cutting, coagulation, and ablation of soft tissue. The Renuvion system consists of an electrosurgical generator unit, a hand piece, and a supply of helium gas. RF energy is delivered to the hand piece by the generator and used to energize an electrode. When helium gas is passed over the energized electrode, a helium plasma is generated, which allows heat to be applied to tissue in 2 different and distinct ways. First, heat is generated by the actual production of the plasma beam itself through the ionization and rapid neutralization of the helium atoms. Second, because plasmas are very good electrical conductors, a portion of the RF energy used to energize the electrode and generate the plasma passes from the electrode to the patient and heats tissue by passing current

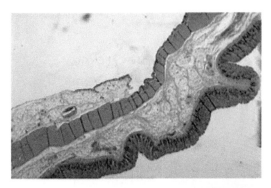

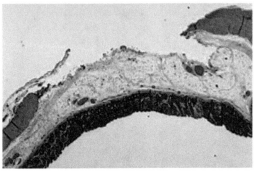

Fig. 7. A demonstration of the wider thermal damage of electrosurgical devices versus CAP/J-Plasma in peritoneum. (*Upper*) Porcine tissue treated with Renuvion/JPlasma. (*Lower*) More extensive tissue thermal damage with standard electocautery. (H&E stains at 100×).

through the resistance of the tissue, a process known as Joule heating. These 2 sources of tissue heating give the Renuvion device some unique advantages during use as a surgical tool for the purpose of coagulation and contraction of subcutaneous soft tissue. These advantages are discussed in more detail later.

Renuvion Instant Tissue Heating Versus Bulk Tissue Heating

Some devices commercially available for subcutaneous soft tissue coagulation work on the principle of bulk tissue heating. In these devices, the energy is primarily directed into the dermis, and the device is activated until a preset subdermal temperature in the range of 65°C is achieved and maintained across the entire volume of tissue. As discussed earlier, at 65°C, the tissue being treated must be maintained at that temperature for greater than 120 seconds for maximal contraction to occur. Although these devices have proven effective in achieving soft tissue contraction,[32] the process of heating all the tissue to the treatment temperature and maintaining that temperature for extended periods can be time consuming. In addition, during this process, the heat eventually

conducts to the epidermis, requiring constant monitoring of epidermal temperatures to ensure they do not exceed safe levels.

A study conducted on a live porcine model to establish the subdermal tissue temperatures produced by the Renuvion device demonstrated a much different philosophy for achieving soft tissue contraction when compared with the commercially available devices described earlier. **Fig. 8** illustrates the methods used in this porcine study. The study simulated actual clinical conditions as closely as possible, including tumescent infiltration and completion of liposuction on the abdomen of the pig. Before beginning treatment with the Renuvion device, an incision was made through the epidermis and dermis into the subdermal plane to serve as a visualization window through which a forward-looking infrared radiometer (FLIR) camera could measure internal tissue temperatures. Multiple treatment passes of the Renuvion device were then conducted using a matrix of various treatment combinations. For each treatment combination tested, a single treatment pass consisted of 3 strokes of the device in the subdermal plane (see **Fig. 8**). The second treatment stroke was performed so that the tip of the Renuvion device passed directly underneath the visualization window. This novel testing method allowed the FLIR camera to capture both internal and external tissue temperatures simultaneously. **Fig. 9** shows an example of the images captured by the FLIR camera as the device passes under the visualization window. Typical results from the porcine study are shown in **Fig. 10**. It is important to note that the time shown on the x-axis in this graph is reported in milliseconds.

The Renuvion device heats the tissue to temperatures greater than 85°C for between 0.040 and 0.080 seconds[33] (see **Fig. 10**). Heating the tissue to these temperatures for this period of time is adequate for achieving maximal soft tissue coagulation and contraction. However, unlike with bulk tissue heating, the tissue surrounding the treatment site remains at much cooler temperatures, resulting in rapid cooling after the application of the energy through conductive heat transfer. In addition, the energy from the Renuvion system is focused on heating the fibroseptal network (FSN) instead of the dermis. Published studies have shown that most soft tissue contraction induced by subcutaneous energy delivery devices is due to its effect on the FSN.[34,35] Because of these unique heating and cooling properties of the Renuvion technology, immediate soft tissue contraction can be achieved without unnecessarily heating the full thickness of the dermis.

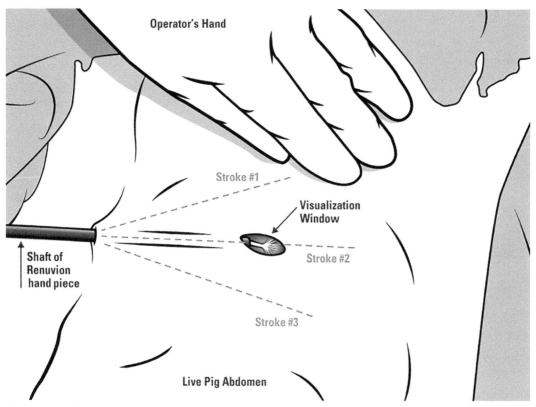

Fig. 8. Methods used in tissue temperature study.

Renuvion 360° Tissue Treatment

It is known that electrical energy takes the path of least resistance. As discussed earlier, RF energy flows through the conductive plasma beam generated by the Renuvion system. This conductive plasma beam can be thought of as a flexible wire or electrode that "connects" to the tissue that represents the path of least resistance for the flow of the RF energy. Tissue that represents the path of least resistance is typically either the tissue that is in closest proximity to the tip of

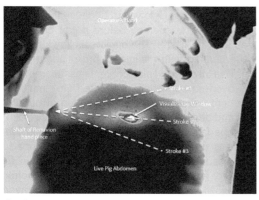

Fig. 9. FLIR camera image.

the Renuvion device or the tissue that has the lowest impedance (is the easiest to pass energy through). When used for the coagulation of subcutaneous soft tissue, this means that the energy from the Renuvion device is not directed or focused in any set direction when activated in the subdermal plane as in some RFAL devices. If the path of least resistance is through the overlying dermis, the plasma energy will be directed to the dermis. If the path of least resistance is through the FSN, the plasma energy will be directed there. As the tip of the Renuvion device is drawn through the subdermal plane, new structures are introduced to the tip of the device, and the path of least resistance is constantly changing. As the energy is constantly finding a new preferred path, the plasma beam quickly alternates between treating the different tissue surrounding the tip of the device. The flow of energy in this device allows for 360° tissue treatment without the need for the user to redirect the flow of energy. Because the FSN is typically the closest tissue to the tip of the Renuvion device, most of the energy delivered by the device results in coagulation and contraction of the fibroseptal bands. Maximizing the energy flow to the FSN expedites the soft tissue contraction process.

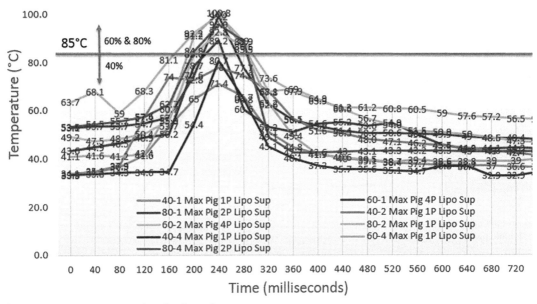

Fig. 10. Temperature versus time for Renuvion treatment.

Renuvion: Consistent Power Output

The design of the electrosurgical generator for the Renuvion plasma device is fundamentally different from monopolar and bipolar devices. As shown in the "Output Power versus Impedance Curves" in **Fig. 11**, monopolar and bipolar devices have limited power output in tissues with higher impedance, such as fat. The Renuvion device was designed to maintain consistent power output over a wide range of impedances. When used for the coagulation of subdermal tissue, the Renuvion output is not self-limiting and provides unencumbered delivery of power regardless of the tissue impedance.

Renuvion: Minimal Depth of Thermal Effect

Not all RF energy is created equal. Experienced RF users know that one can achieve very different tissue results at the same power setting by simply changing from an RF waveform designed for cutting to an RF waveform designed for coagulation. The proprietary waveform of the Renuvion device has much lower current than typical monopolar RF devices. In most cases, the current of the Renuvion device is an order of magnitude lower. As discussed earlier, the current of the Renuvion waveform flows through the conductive plasma beam to create additional beneficial Joule heating of the target tissue. However, because the current is so low, it is dispersed before it can penetrate deep into the tissue. The dispersal allows for soft tissue heating with minimal depth of thermal effect. This low current also prevents tissue from being overtreated when subjected to multiple treatment passes. As tissue is treated, it coagulates and desiccates, resulting in an increase in tissue impedance. The lower current of the Renuvion device is unable to push through higher impedance tissue. As the Renuvion device passes in proximity to previously treated tissue, the energy will follow the path of least resistance (lower impedance) and preferentially treat previously

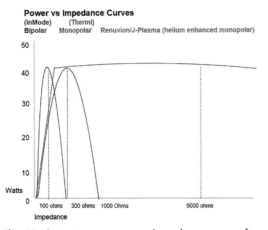

Fig. 11. Output power versus impedance curves for subdermal energy devices.

untreated tissue. This prevents overtreating of any one area with multiple passes and maximizes the treatment of untreated tissue.

Renuvion: Helium

Although other inert gases can and have been used in plasma devices for medical applications, the Renuvion device uses helium because of its unique properties, which translate into certain clinical advantages. Helium has a simple molecular structure consisting of only 2 electrons. This simple structure allows helium to be ionized using very low input of energy. The ionization of helium is therefore very controlled and produces a precise and stable output of energy. Helium facilitates the use of the low-current, proprietary RF waveform from the Renuvion generator.

In summary, the Renuvion helium-based plasma device from BMC has technological features that result in a unique and effective method of action for subdermal coagulation and contraction of soft tissue. These features are as follows:

1. The Renuvion device achieves soft tissue coagulation and contraction by rapidly heating the treatment site to temperatures greater than 85°C for between 0.040 and 0.080 seconds.[33]
2. The tissue surrounding the treatment site remains at much cooler temperatures, resulting in rapid cooling after the application of the energy through conductive heat transfer.
3. The creation of a gaseous subdermal environment (helium) re-creates atmospheric-like pressures, which exist with cutaneous treatments and helps to dissipate accumulated thermal energy.
4. Focused delivery of energy is on immediate heating of the FSN, resulting in immediate soft tissue contraction without unnecessarily heating the full thickness of the dermis.
5. Tissue treatment is 360° without the need for the user to redirect the flow of energy due to electrical energy taking the path of least resistance.
6. Unencumbered delivery of power is regardless of the tissue impedance due to the unique power output from the electrosurgical generator.
7. Low-current RF energy results in minimal depth of thermal effect and prevention of overtreating tissue when performing multiple passes.

RENUVION FOR SKIN TIGHTENING AND SKIN REJUVENATION

Laser, RF, high-frequency focused ultrasound, and other thermal-induced contractions of collagen are well known in medicine and are used in ophthalmology, orthopedic applications, and the treatment of varicose veins. Each type of collagen has an optimal contraction temperature that does not cause thermal destruction of connective tissue, but induces a restructuring effect in collagen fibers. The reported range of temperatures causing collagen shrinkage varies from 60°C to 85°C.[34] At this temperature, tissue contraction occurs immediately after tissue reaches the threshold temperature. The shrinkage of tissue is dramatic and can reach up to 30% of the heated tissue volume. This type of contraction is well studied in cornea, joints, cartilage, and vascular tissue, but its application for skin, subdermal tissue, and subcutaneous tissue tightening has been rarely studied.[34] Noninvasive tissue tightening treatments have an inherent safety limitation because energy is delivered through the skin surface, and the threshold epidermal burn temperature is significantly lower than the optimal temperature for the collagen contraction. Studies indicate that deeper penetrating energy provides better skin contraction, and RF energy, by penetrating deeper than laser radiation, is a superior method, not only for treatment of facial rhytids and laxity but also for body tightening. When considering skin contraction, 2-dimensional horizontal x-axis tightening of the skin surface must be differentiated from 3-dimensional x-y-z tissue tightening of the subcutaneous tissue, where the skin is also more firmly connected and adjacent to the deeper anatomic structures. If 2-dimensional contraction is a function of collagen structure changes in the dermis, the 3-dimensional tissue-tightening changes involve contraction of different types of collagenous tissue. The following types of collagen tissue can be separated in the subcutaneous space:

- Dermis: papillary and reticular
- Fascia: Relatively thick layer of connective tissue located between muscles and skin
- Septal connective tissue: Thin layers of connective tissue separating lobules of fat and connecting dermis with fascia
- Reticular fibers: Framework of single collagen fibers encasing fat cells[34]

The authors agree with Kenkel[36] that skin tightening and elasticity changes following thermal injury of soft tissues, including fat and collagen, are mostly a result of subdermal tissue contraction, but not dermal contraction only, which experiences lower heating during the treatment. It is clear that 40°C to 42°C applied to the skin surface cannot result in an immediate contraction effect. Deep dermal remodeling may account for some horizontal contraction over time. It is possible that the dermal-fat junction experiences higher temperatures, but this process requires future investigation. Most of the thinking on this is that the mechanism of subcutaneous collagen contraction during thermal stimulation of the interstitial space is like that witnessed in other types of collagen in that the contraction process has thermal contraction thresholds in the range of 60°C to 70°C. It is likely more accurate to talk about tissue contraction rather than skin tightening because significant area contraction is a result of the strong contribution of deeper adipose fascial layers. Further studies with accurate 3-dimensional area measurements will tell more about thermal-mediated technology. These thermal processes and contraction can be effectively applied during different microinvasive surgical procedures, improving patient satisfaction and extending procedures like facial and body contouring procedures to higher-weight patients and patients with compromised skin conditions.[35] Skin rejuvenation results with CAP/J-Plasma have been very impressive. The high temperatures applied at the epidermis and extending into the dermis and possible deeper penetration to the FSN result in a level of rhytid correction that is seen only with the most ablative skin rejuvenation devices: full-face ablative carbon dioxide and full-face phenol or trichloroacetic acid face peelings. Although the results from this treatment can be dramatic, the prolonged recovery issues remain the same and that is the propensity for prolonged erythema. The authors are currently working on recovery protocols to lessen the erythema because the results for skin rejuvenation from this device are unsurpassed.

Case Study 1: Renuvion/J-Plasma Skin Tightening/Rejuvenation

This 59-year-old female presented for facial rejuvenation. During her consultation we discussed with her the volume depleted status of her skin and significant actinic sun damage. Rather than proceed with a surgical approach we decided to perform Renuvion Skin Rejuvenation with both micro and nanofat grafting to entire face. About 50 cc of fat were transferred (**Fig. 12**).

RENUVION/J-PLASMA FOR RHINOPHYMA TREATMENT

Rhinophyma is a skin disorder characterized by a large, red, bumpy, or bulbous nose. It can occur as part of phymatous rosacea. The exact cause of rhinophyma is unknown, but it is considered a subtype of severe rosacea. Overall, rosacea is a common, chronic inflammatory skin condition. Although the ravages of subtype 3 (phymatous) rosacea have been well documented throughout history, today, a multitude of options are available to restore a red, swollen, or bumpy nose (rhinophyma) to normal appearance. Although rosacea was not identified as a distinct medical disorder until the early twentieth century, its existence has long been recorded in arts and literature, from the bumpy nose of the "Old Man and a Boy" by Ghirlandaio in 1490, a vivid representation of rhinophyma, to the red faces of subtype 1 rosacea depicted in "Dutch Merrymakers at Shrovetide," by Frans Hals in 1617.

Early candid photographs show that the famed financier J.P. Morgan was afflicted with rhinophyma, including one in which he is brandishing an umbrella or walking stick to discourage the photographer, because his official picture was altered to correct the image of his nose, according to an article by Drs Warren Dotz and Neil Berliner.[37] Severe rhinophyma may be treated with surgical therapy, including lasers, cryosurgery, RF ablation, electrosurgery, a heated scalpel, electrocautery, and tangential excision, combined with scissor sculpting, skin grafting, or dermabrasion. Often a CO_2 or erbium:YAG laser may be used as a bloodless scalpel to remove excess tissue and recontour the nose to a normal appearance, and fractional resurfacing may be of value in mild cases. To this list of treatment entities, the authors would add the CAP/J-Plasma ablation, and this will most likely become the superior treatment modality for several reasons. Other treatment modalities have suggested high-frequency electrosurgery for shaving of subtype 3 (phymatous) rhinophyma.[38] The dual cutting and vaporizing capabilities of the CAP/J-Plasma device make it ideal for treating severe rhinophyma. The retractable blade serves as a sculpting device and will operate with more thermal precision (less collateral thermal damage) in removing diseased tissue. After major debulking with the blade, the blade is retracted, and fine tuning of the rhinophyma is achieved with microplasma. The helium-based gas plasma surgical technology that powers J-Plasma takes much of the heat out of surgery. Although J-Plasma turns down the heat, it ups the precision to micron level. It safely removes tissue cells layer by layer, allowing surgeons to ablate the affected tissue by "painting," a technique that spares the healthy tissue that lies beneath. It is the authors' opinion that the CAP/J-Plasma device will become the treatment

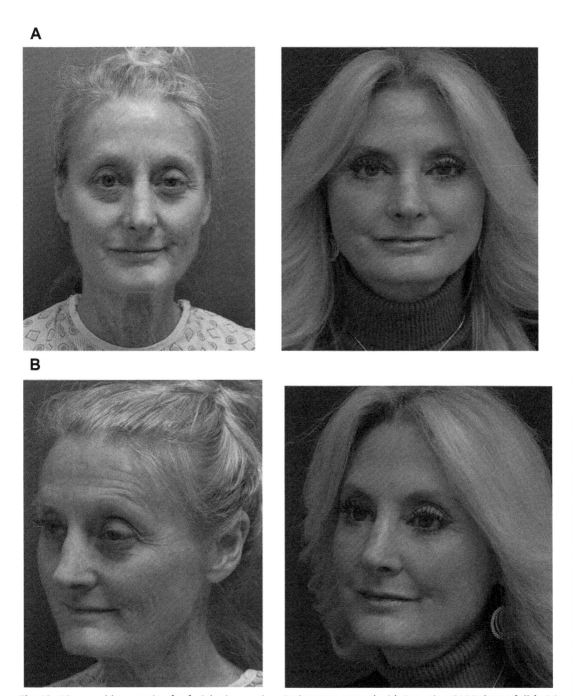

Fig. 12. 59-year-old presenting for facial rejuvenation. Patient was treated with Renuvion CAP/Jplasma full facial and down to mandibular border and the neck was peeled with 25% TCA. Microfat grafting and nanofat grafting was done to the entire face and lip creases (50cc total). Patient show before and three months after procedure. (*A*) Frontal before and after and (*B*) oblique lateral before and after. Interestingly her left eye ptosis showed some improvement from the skin tightening inherent with the Renuvion treatment.

of choice for hypertrophic thickened subtype 3 (phymatous) rhinophyma. In addition to the precise shaving and vaporization capabilities, the device also exerts a high antibacterial effect, and as discussed previously, CAP appear to possess antineoplastic capabilities, which sometimes accompany advanced rhinophyma. The antibacterial effects also will play a part for future development of device strategies to treat biofilms of all causes.

Case Study 2: Renuvion/J-Plasma Treatment of Phymatous Rhinophyma

The patient presented with severe subtype 3 (phymatous) rhinophyma and nasal obstruction and with cosmetic concerns about his enlarged nose.[21] The patient underwent successful treatment with CAP/J-Plasma and is shown before and 10 weeks after treatment[39] (**Fig. 13**).

RENUVION/J-PLASMA FOR MINIMALLY INVASIVE JOWL SUBMENTAL AND NECK TIGHTENING

Less invasive procedures for facial rejuvenation are becoming more popular as prospective patients seek out treatment options that offer the best possible results with the least amount of downtime. As the demand for "quick recovery" procedures increases and patients spend more time researching options, more informed choices are being made, and many times patients opt for technologically advanced procedures. Such has been the case with the evolution of fiber laser, temperature-controlled RF, and ultrasound-based techniques in a genre of subdermal surgical techniques now termed "thermoplastic rejuvenation."[40–47] This class of energy-based devices used subdermally now includes plasma devices.[48] The procedures developed are now commonly termed "nonexcisional" facial rejuvenation and can be performed with many different types of technologies. Non-excisional procedures aim to produce lipolysis and fat reduction in the areas affected, particularly the jowl and submentum, and to tighten collagen and soft tissue in the adjacent FSN and in the dermis. These associated changes create both facial contouring of the heavy face and neck, and also provide skin tightening for additional benefit. The thermal precision found in CAP/J-Plasma has some advantages over laser or temperature-controlled RF. The device-tissue interface is selectively treated by the high-energy microplasma, but leaves the subdermal region and the nerve-bearing regions relatively unaffected. This lack of thermal penetration is encouraging with respect to patient safety and comfort, but it may require more passes than other technologies because of limited thermal effects of the CAP/J-Plasma.

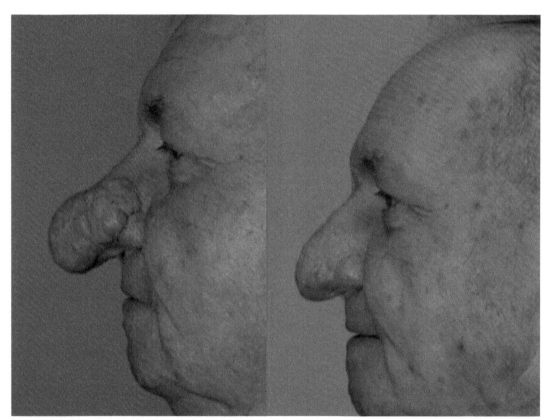

Fig. 13. Patient with phymatous rhinophyma shown before and 10 weeks after rhinophyma thinning/ablation with CAP/J-Plasma. (*Left*) Before treatment. (*Right*) After treatment with Renuvion/JPlasma. (*Courtesy of* Ali Tehrani, DO, Apple Valley, CA.)

Case Study 3: Renuvion/J-Plasma Microinvasive and Nonexcisional Treatment of Lower Face and Neck

The patient is a 52-year-old woman interested in a nonexcisional procedure that would help with loose skin at the corners of the mouth as well as address jowl heaviness and submental fullness. She is treated with subcutaneous Renuvion via submental incision and lobular puncture incision and is shown before and 3 months after her procedure. Additional tightening and definition should occur for up 6 months and to a lesser extent 1 year. Micro-liposuction is also done in conjunction with these procedures using a 2-mm cannula. Subplatysmal dissection was done with the device, and limited platysmaplasty was performed as well. A more defined mandibular contour is shown afterward with slimming of the lower face and submentum. The mandibular cervical and submental angles are significantly improved (**Fig. 14**).

Case Study 4 Renuvion/J-Plasma Microinvasive and Nonexcisional Treatment of Neck

The patient is a 50-year-old woman who dislikes the loss of her cervicofacial contour with the accumulation of excess submental fat. She is treated with subcutaneous Renuvion via submental incision and lobular puncture incision and is shown before and 3 months after her procedure. Additional tightening and definition should occur for up 6 months and to a lesser extent for 1 year. Micro-liposuction is also done in conjunction with these procedures using a 2-mm cannula. Subplatysmal dissection was done with the device, and limited platysmaplasty was performed as well. As in case study 3, a more defined mandibular contour is shown afterward with slimming of the lower face and submentum. The mandibular cervical and submental angles are significantly improved (**Fig. 15**).

RENUVION/J-PLASMA OTHER APPLICATIONS

Renuvion has been used for rhytidectomy and is helpful in elevating flaps, and especially, in ligamentous release of the mandibular and zygomatic ligaments. The thermal dynamics of the technology permit precise elevation of flaps without potential added thermal damage of the dermal plexus of vessels above the subcutaneous plane or below where most nerves reside. The blade feature facilitates easy subcutaneous dissection, not only in the face but also in the neck.

The authors have also used Renuvion for skin tightening after laser lipolysis and for improvement of cellulite.

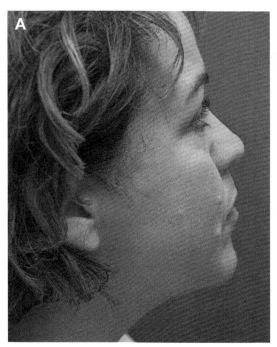 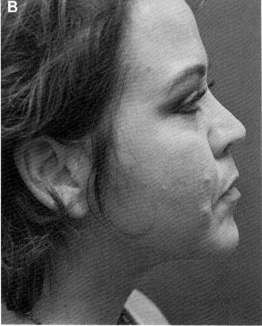

Fig. 14. The patient is a 52-year-old who dislikes the loss of contour in mandible and submentum. She is shown (*A*) before and (*B*) 3 months after nonexcisional facial and neck contouring using CAP/J-Plasma. Improvement in jawline and submentum is evident. Treatment included the lower face.

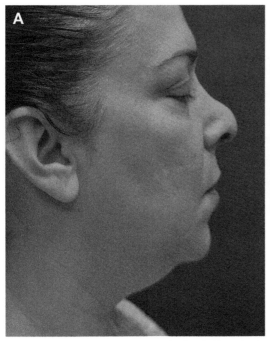
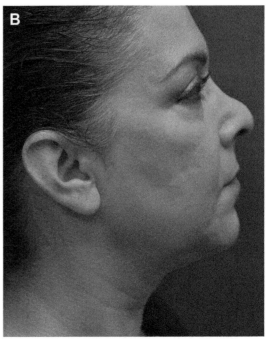

Fig. 15. The patient is a 52-year-old who dislikes the loss of contour in mandible and submentum. She is shown (*A*) before and (*B*) 3 months after nonexcisional facial and neck contouring using CAP/J-Plasma. Improvement in jawline and submentum is evident. The treatment in this patient did not include the lower face.

COMPLICATIONS

Patients treated with Renuvion usually will not incur more or different complications than listed as potential complications for the procedure being performed. In fact, compared with other energy-based devices used in the subcutaneous or interstitial space, such as fiber lasers or RF devices, whether temperature controlled or not, the complication profile is relatively less, and this is due to the volume of unionized helium gas under the flaps, which serves as a concurrent air conditioner. The thermal profile of Renuvion combined with the unionized helium gas provides a more balanced environment than the energy-based devices acting alone. One must be cautious to not use excessive energy in the fascial planes because this can be associated with an increased incidence of seroma formation. The authors have seen no skin burns or skin necrosis associated with the subdermal use of Renuvion in more than 100 procedures to date.

SUMMARY

Renuvion/J-Plasma offers unique benefits compared with CO_2 laser and conventional electrosurgical devices, including the following:

- Enhanced clinical effects
- No complicated setup or safety procedures

- No credentialing/certification required
- No additional insurance requirements

Renuvion/J-Plasma is an advanced energy device combining the unique properties of CHP with RF energy. Helium plasma focuses RF energy for greater control of tissue effect, enabling a high level of precision and virtually eliminating unintended tissue trauma.

Renuvion key benefits include low risk of injury to surrounding tissue due to the following:

- Minimized lateral and depth of thermal spread;
- Plasma stream length controllable and precise at the micron level;
- Less smoke, odor, and eschar;
- No conductive currents through the patients;
- Effectiveness on many tissue types.

The Renuvion retractable blade enables greater versatility and control of the energy as well as enhanced visibility at the application site. Pistol-grip and pencil hand pieces with single-button cutting, dissection, ablation and coagulation.

Cool helium plasma offers unique benefits compared with CO_2 laser, including the following:

- Enhanced clinical effects
- No complicated setup or safety procedures

- No credentialing/certification required
- No additional insurance requirements

Renuvion offers many advantages for facial plastic surgeons in performing surgeries, such as rhinophyma reduction, skin tightening and rejuvenation, microinvasive, and nonexcisional facial and neck rejuvenation, and may also be helpful in treating skin cancers. The authors are optimistic that these devices will provide technology that improves and enhances patient care into the future.

REFERENCES

1. Feldman LS, Fuchshuber PR, Jones DB. The SAGES manual on the fundamental use of surgical energy (FUSE). Berlin/Heidelberg (Germany): Springer Science+Business Media, LLC; 2012.
2. Menashi WP. Treatment of surfaces. U.S. Patent 3383163. 1968.
3. GutBoucher RM. Seeded gas plasma sterilization method. U.S.Patent 4 207 286. 1980.
4. Jacobs PT, Lin SM. Hydogen peroxide plasma sterilization system. U.S. Patent 4 643 876. 1987.
5. Gitomer SJ, Jones RD. Laser-produced plasmas in medicine. IEEE Trans Plasma Sci 1991;19(6): 1209–19.
6. Laroussi M. Low-temperature plasma jet for biomedical applications: a review. IEEE Trans Plasma Sci 2015;43:703–12.
7. Koinuma H, Ohkubo H, Hashimoto T, et al. Development and application of a microbeam plasma generator. Appl Phys Lett 1992;3(7):816–7.
8. Inomata K, Ha H, Chaudhary KA, et al. Open air deposition of SiO_2 film from a cold plasma torch of tetramethoxysilane-H_2-Ar system. Appl Phys Lett 1994;3:46.
9. Ha H, Inomata K, Koinuma H. Plasma chemical vapor deposition of SiO2 on air-exposed surfaces by cold plasma torch. J Electrochem Soc 1995;3(8): 2726–30.
10. Inomata K, Koinuma H, Oikawa Y, et al. Open air photoresist ashing by a cold plasma torch: catalytic effect of cathode material. Appl Phys Lett 1995;3: 2188.
11. Ha H, Yoshimoto M, Koinuma H, et al. Open air plasma chemical vapor deposition of highly dielectric amorphous TiO_2 films. Appl Phys Lett 1996;3: 2965.
12. Ha H, Moon BK, Horiuchi T, et al. Structure and electric properties of TiO2 films prepared by cold plasma torch under atmospheric pressure. Mater Sci Eng 1996;3(1):143–7.
13. Inomata K, Aoki N, Koinuma H. Jpn J Appl Phys 1994;197.
14. Lee B, Kusano Y, Kato N, et al. Oxygen plasma treatment of rubber surface by the atmospheric pressure cold plasma torch. Jpn J Appl Phys 1997;3(5A): 2888–91.
15. Stoffels E, Flikweert AJ, Stoffels WW, et al. Plasma needle: a non–destructive atmospheric plasma source for fine surface treatment of (bio) materials. Plasma Sources Sci T 2002;3:383–8.
16. Kieft IE, Laan EP, Stoffels E. Electrical and optical characterization of the plasma needle. New J Phys 2004;3:149.
17. Li SZ, Huang WT, Zhang J, et al. Optical diagnosis of an argon/oxygen needle plasma generated at atmospheric pressure. Appl Phys Lett 2009;3: 111501.
18. Gumbel D, Bekeschus S, Gelbrich N, et al. Cold atmospheric plasma in the treatment of osteosarcoma. Int J Mol Sci 2017;18(9):2004.
19. Yan D, Sherman JH, Keidar M. Cold atmospheric plasma, a novel promising anti-cancer treatment modality. Oncotarget 2017;8:15977–95.
20. Pedroso JP, Gutierrez M, Volker W. Thermal effect of JPlasma energy in a porcine tissue model: implications for minimally invasive surgery. Available at: http://www.boviemedical.com/wp-content/uploads/2016/06/WP-Thermal_Effect_Of-J-Plasma_Energy_In_A_Porcine_Tissue_Model_Implications_For_Minimally_Invasive_Surgery.pdf. Accessed November 2018.
21. Goldberg SN, Gazelle GS, Halpern EF, et al. Radiofrequency tissue ablation: importance of local temperature along the electrode tip exposure in determining lesion shape and size. Acad Radiol 1996;3:212–8.
22. Thomsen S. Pathologic analysis of photothermal and photomechanical effects of laser-tissue interactions. Photochem Photobiol 1991;53:825–35.
23. Ross EV, McKinlay JR, Anderson RR. Why does carbon dioxide resurfacing work? A review. Arch Dermatol 1999;135(4):444–54.
24. Gardner ES, Reinisch L, Stricklin GP, et al. In vitro changes in non-facial human skin following CO2 laser resurfacing: a comparison study. Lasers Surg Med 1996;19(4):379–87.
25. Chen SS, Wright NT, Humphrey JD. Heat-induced changes in the mechanics of a collagenous tissue: isothermal free shrinkage. J Biomech Eng 1997; 109:372–8.
26. Doshi SN, Alster TS. Combination radiofrequency and diode laser for treatment of facial rhytides and skin laxity. J Cosmet Laser Ther 2005;7:11–5.
27. Fatemi A, Weiss MA, Weiss RA. Short-term histologic effects of nonablative resurfacing: results with a dynamically cooled millisecond-domain 1320nm Nd:YAG laser. Dermatol Surg 2002;28(2): 172–6.
28. Mayoral FA. Skin tightening with a combined unipolar and bipolar radiofrequency device. J Drugs Dermatol 2007;6(2):212–5.

29. Alster TS, Doshi SN, Hpping SB. Combination surgical lifting with ablative laser skin resurfacing of facial skin: a retrospective analysis. Dermatol Surg 2004; 30(9):1191–5.

30. Zelickson B, Kist D, Bernstein E, et al. Histological and ultrastructural evaluation of the effects of a radiofrequency-based nonablative dermal remodeling device: a pilot study. Arch Dermatol 2004;140: 204–9.

31. Hsu T, Kaminer M. The use of nonablative radiofrequency technology to tighten the lower face and neck. Semin Cutan Med Surg 2003;22:115–23.

32. Duncan DI. Nonexcisional tissue tightening: creating skin surface area reduction during abdominal liposuction by adding radiofrequency heating. Aesthet Surg J 2013;33(8):1154–66.

33. Technical brief: internal and external tissue temperature in subdermal coagulation. Bovie Medical Corporation; 2018. MM0154.00 0718.

34. Paul M, Blugerman G, Kreindel M, et al. Three-dimensional radiofrequency tissue tightening: a proposed mechanism and applications for body contouring. Aesthetic Plast Surg 2011;35(1):87–95.

35. Hurwitz D, Smith D. Treatment of overweight patients by radiofrequency-assisted liposuction (RFAL) for aesthetic reshaping and skin tightening. Aesthetic Plast Surg 2012;36(1):62–71.

36. Kenkel JM. Evaluation of skin tightening after laser-assisted liposuction, commentary. Plast Reconstr Surg 2009;29(5):407–40.

37. Dotz W, Berliner N. Rhinophyma: a master's depiction, a patron's affliction. Am J Dermatopathol 1984;6:231–5.

38. Aferzon M, Millman B. Excision of rhinophyma with high-frequency electrosurgery. Dermatol Surg 2002;28(8):735–8.

39. Available at: www.boviemedical.com/wp-content/.../J-Plasma_Rhinophyma_Feature_Story.pdf. Accessed October 18, 2017.

40. Gentile RD. Smartlifting ™-A technological Innovation for facial rejuvenation. Cynosure white paper Available at: http://3te441c5la742885k7f5ybi8.wpengine.netdna-cdn.com/wp-content/uploads/2013/06/smartlipo_triplex_compendium.pdf. pp22-25. Accessed October 16, 2017.

41. Gentile RD. Smartlifting ™-A technological innovation for facial rejuvenation. Lasers Surg Med 2009; 41(Supplement 21).

42. Gentile RD. LaserFacialSculpting™ minimally invasive techniques for facial rejuvenation utilizing the Smartlipo™ Nd:YAG laser February 1, 2010. Available at: http://66.36.229.213/live/cynosureapp/Smartlipo_MPX_TP/smartlook_smartlifting/921-0187-000_r2_LaserFacialSculptingWP.pdf. Accessed April 27, 2014.

43. Gentile RD. SmartLifting™ fiber laser-assisted facial rejuvenation techniques. Facial Plast Surg Clin North Am 2011;19(2):371–87.

44. Gentile RD. Laser-assisted neck-lift: high-tech contouring and tightening. Facial Plast Surg 2011; 27(4):331–45.

45. Gentile RD. Subcutaneous fiber laser and energy-based techniques for facial rejuvenation. In: Truswell WH, editor. Lasers and light peels and abrasions. New York: Thieme publishers; 2016.

46. Kinney BM, Andriessen A, DiBernardo BE, et al. Use of a controlled subdermal radio frequency thermistor for treating the aging neck: consensus recommendations. J Cosmet Laser Ther 2017; 19(8):444–50.

47. Gentile RD, Kinney BM, Sadick NS. Radiofrequency technology in face and neck rejuvenation [review]. Facial Plast Surg Clin North Am 2018; 26(2):123–34.

48. Gentile RD. Cool atmospheric Plasma (J-Plasma®) and new options for facial contouring and skin rejuvenation of the heavy face and neck [review]. Facial Plast Surg 2018;34(1): 66–74.

Radiofrequency Microneedling
Overview of Technology, Advantages, Differences in Devices, Studies, and Indications

Steven F. Weiner, MD

KEYWORDS

- Radiofrequency • RF Microneedling • Fractional RF • Highintensity RF • Microneedling • Laxity
- Neck rejuvenation • Acne scarring

KEY POINTS

- RF skin rejuvenation is improved using RF microneedling devices. More aggressive treatments are performed safely with minimal downtime than previous RF devices.
- Optimizing treatment parameters is essential for safety and efficacy.
- Multiple RFM studies support minimal risks even in dark skin types.
- RFM has been used to treat acne scarring successfully as well as skin laxity and hyperhidrosis.

HISTORY OF RADIOFREQUENCY

The use of radiofrequency (RF) in medicine is ubiquitous and dates back over 75 years. Energy produced from RF has been used for cautery of tissues/vessels, tightening of pharyngeal tissues in sleep apnea, and to destroy tumors. RF is used to ablate accessory conduction pathways in the heart to improve atrial fibrillation and other conditions. RF diathermy is used in occupational and physical therapy to apply heat to deeper tissues. The term "radiofrequency" originates from the frequency of the electricity used is similar to that of radio waves.

In 2002, ThermaCool became the first RF device approved for cosmetic use (periocular rhytids) and, in 2004, it received approval for treatment of facial wrinkles and rhytids. In 2006, off face use was approved. Dozens of RF devices have since been approved for esthetic use with various methods used to deliver the energy to the dermis and fibroseptal network in the subcutaneous fat.

TYPES OF RADIOFREQUENCY

There are 2 different delivery mechanisms which RF uses: monopolar and bipolar.

Monopolar RF: the energy flows from an active electrode within the operator's handpiece to a grounding pad (passive electrode) placed distally on the patient's body. Early RF devices (ThermaCool) used monopolar RF, and it is still a popular technology in current devices. Its advantage is that the energy can be deposited rather deeply from a surface electrode-deep dermis and fibroseptal network.

Bipolar RF: the energy flows between 2 adjacent electrodes, both contained within the operator's handpiece. The depth of penetration (for the transepidermal devices) is postulated to approximate half the distance between the electrodes, although this is not universally accepted.[1] Higher energies can be delivered with bipolar than monopolar, but the depths are less.

Disclosure Statement: Lutronic-Infini, Carestream-Pronox.
2050 West County Highway 30A, Suite 114, Santa Rosa Beach, FL 32459, USA
E-mail address: info@theclinique.net

Facial Plast Surg Clin N Am 27 (2019) 291–303
https://doi.org/10.1016/j.fsc.2019.03.002
1064-7406/19/

RADIOFREQUENCY ENERGY DELIVERY

Radiofrequency creates oscillating electrical current (millions of cycles per second), causing vibration and collisions between charged molecules, thus resulting in production of heat, as described by Belenky and colleagues[2] Electrical energy is converted to thermal energy as resistance in the tissue is met.[3] Energy transfer is dictated by Ohm's Law: energy (J) = $I^2 \times R \times T$ (where I is the current, R is the tissue impedance, and T is the time of application). Impendence depends on skin hydration, electrolyte composition, collagen content, temperature, and other variables.[4] Unlike lasers, which use a photothermal energy (selective photothermolysis), RF energy is independent of pigmentation/skin type, and is strictly an electrothermal effect. The RF devices used in esthetic procedures range from 0.3 to 10 MHz. Depth of penetration is inversely proportional to frequency used.[5]

RADIOFREQUENCY: EARLY APPLICATIONS AND DEFICIENCIES

The initial RF devices pushed energy through the epidermis to the deeper layers using monopolar technology. However, the depth of the heating is not precise and there are cases of fat destruction from inadvertent subdermal heating.[6] There are also limitations in the temperatures that the epidermis can handle to avoid complications such as postinflammatory hyperpigmentation (PIH), blistering, and scarring. It has been noted that maintaining the skin surface to temperatures below 42°C to 45°C is essential for safe RF treatments because the threshold for epidermal burn is 44°C. The methods for which devices have used to overcome epidermal heating problems have been superficial cooling and constant motion of the handpiece. To cool the skin, cryogen spray or a cooling plate is applied to the skin simultaneously with the energy pulse and leads to a reverse temperature gradient—deeper tissues achieving higher temperatures.[7]

By delivering energy through a constantly moving RF energy handpiece, the skin heating can be more gradual and safer. Temperature can be monitored either by sensors within the handpiece or with an infrared camera. Treatment is either paused or completed when the surface temperature reaches 42°C to 45°C. The downside to this technique is that the provider can fatigue during the treatment or during subsequent procedures later in the day. Uniform heating might not be achieved under these circumstances.

Bulk heating occurs with these superficial RF devices, which means the epidermis, dermis, fibroseptal network, and adnexa are all heated simultaneously, albeit to different temperatures. Heat accumulation is longer, as dissipation is slowed when an entire area is heated versus a "fractional heating" technique. Leaving unaffected tissue adjacent to treated areas creates more rapid healing and safer treatments for lasers and RF.

Transepidermal RF tissue tightening treatments have an inherent limitation because energy is delivered through the skin surface and the threshold to prevent epidermal burns is significantly lower than the optimal temperature for neocollagenesis. Whereas there are mild benefits to heating of the dermis to 45°C to 60°C to get partial collagen denaturing, optimal results can be achieved only when dermal temperatures reach 65°C to 70°C, when coagulation and collagen denaturing occurs. At these levels, collagen removal and replacement occurs.[8,9] Biopsies have shown no increases in fibroblast numbers with lower energy levels (below coagulation temperatures), and only collagen thickening/contraction. In contrast, higher-energy levels have shown to result in a hyperplastic response and increases in cellularity during the wound healing response, which continued for 10 weeks or longer.[10] Attempts have been made to deliver higher temperatures to the dermis with the transepidermal RF devices using small, high-energy (concentrated) handpieces, but these have led to epidermal injuries[11] (**Fig. 1**).

WHY RADIOFREQUENCY MICRONEEDLING VERSUS LASERS

In the early 1990s, ablative lasers were introduced and showed marked results in reversing the aging skin of the face. Unfortunately, these lasers had prolonged downtime, and high complication rates[12] (persistent erythema, hypopigmentation, infection, and scarring) and they fell out of favor in the early 2000s. Nonablative lasers were introduced with less downtime and risks, but results did not match the ablative lasers and multiple treatments were needed. Fractional technology was introduced in the mid-2000s initially with nonablative lasers and later with ablative lasers. Ablative lasers came back in favor because the risks and downtime were reduced when healthy tissue surrounding the ablated areas sped up healing.[13,14]

Despite advances in lasers, there remains 2 deficiencies. Because the heat affects the epidermis and dermis with a temperature gradient highest at the skin surface, darker skin types remain at risk for PIH. Measures to reduce PIH are pretreatment

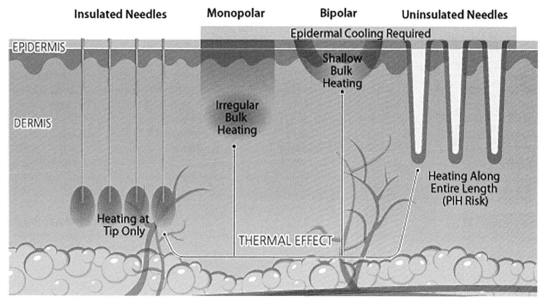

Fig. 1. Heating patterns of various RF delivery devices. (*Courtesy of* Lutronic, Billerica, MA.)

and posttreatment hydroquinone, tretinoin, and skin cooling (during the procedure) but these do not eliminate the problem.[14]

The other problem with lasers has been neck rejuvenation. Owing to the lack of pilosebaceous units, neck healing after deep dermal laser treatments is slowed and impaired. Complication rates of ablative laser treatments of the neck is higher than facial procedures, even when using fractional technology.[15–17]

Radiofrequency has become a viable option for skin rejuvenation and tightening. Using electro-thermal energy versus photothermal energy with lasers, RF is not chromophore dependent and therefore considered applicable for all skin types. This does not equate to meaning that darker skin types are free from risk. Radiofrequency offers little to no downtimes, which is desirable in the current environment of patients' active lifestyles and busy work schedules. Results from transepidermal RF have been highly variable with mostly disappointing results. To further enhance dermal heating, RF microneedling (RFM) was developed. RFM delivers the desired energy through pins/needles that penetrate the skin to a predetermined desired depth. With this technology, dermal heating was improved to the critical level of 65°C to 70°C with epidermal heating minimized when using insulated needles. A reverse thermal gradient is created, with the temperatures highest in the deeper levels, contrasting laser's skin heating. Radiofrequency microneedling overcame the obstacles with laser neck treatment, enabling effective, high-energy delivery without significant downtime or risks. In addition, RFM heat is delivered deeper than laser energy—3 mm or more with certain devices.

INITIAL RADIOFREQUENCY MICRONEEDLING STUDY AND FOLLOW-UP STUDY

The initial study of using RFM was performed by Hantash and colleagues[18] in 2009. Studies were performed on abdominal skin in 15 patients who were later to have abdominoplasty. A handpiece with 5 paired insulated needles with temperature monitoring, and interface feedback with surface cooling was used. Results showed areas of collagen denaturing, RF thermal zone (RTZ) surrounded by areas of normal collagen. Adnexal structures and adipose tissue was spared. No adverse effects were seen.

A follow-up study by Hantash and colleagues[19] in 2009 using a similar novel fractional microneedling RF device showed "A vigorous wound healing response is initiated posttreatment, with a progressive increase in inflammatory cell infiltration from day two through 10 weeks. HSP72 diminished after day 2 while HSP47 increased up to 10 weeks. Increases in IL-1β, TNF-α, and MMP-13 while MMP-1, HSP72, HSP47, and TGF-β levels increased by 2 days. We also observed a marked induction of tropoelastin, fibrillin, as well as procollagens 1 and 3 by 28 days posttreatment. An active dermal remodeling process driven by the collagen chaperone HSP47 leads to complete replacement of RTZs with new collagen by 10 weeks posttreatment. RTZs are observed through day 28 posttreatment but are replaced by new dermal tissue by 10 weeks. Reticular dermal volume, cellularity, HA, and elastin content increase. Furthermore, using immunohistochemical and polymerase chain reaction studies, evidence of profound neoelastinogenesis following RF treatment of human skin is demonstrated. The combination of neoelastinogenesis and neocollagenesis induced by treatment with the fractional microneedling RF system may provide a reliable treatment option for skin laxity and/or rhytids." There is a direct correlation to higher levels of HSP47 and fibroblast proliferation to higher energies delivered.

HISTOLOGY

In a 2014 study by Zheng and colleagues,[20] skin samples that were taken immediately after RFM treatment showed that the RF-induced coagulated columns in the dermis formed a cocoon-shaped zone of subablative thermal injury (**Fig. 2**). Four days after the treatment, skin specimens demonstrated re-epithelialization, and the dermal RF-induced coagulated columns showed mixed cellular infiltration, neovascularization, and granulation tissue formation. Microneedle depth and RF conduction times, but not energy level, significantly affected histometric values of RF-induced dermal coagulation. Microneedle RF treatment affected adnexal structures by coagulating follicular epithelium and perifollicular structures.

Type 1 collagen, the predominant type of collagen in the skin, is composed of a triple-helical polypeptide structure stabilized with crosslinking. The immediate effect of heating is thickening and contraction of the collagen fibers. This is due to destruction of the heat-labile crosslinks of collagen with transformation of the highly organized fiber system into a gel state.[21] Tissue tension in human skin increases because, although the fibers become shorter, the heat-stable crosslinks between molecules are maintained, thus increasing the rubber-elastic properties of the collagen polymer. The heat-modified tissues then undergo remodeling associated with fibroplasia

Intense focused coagulation up to 3.5 mm deep

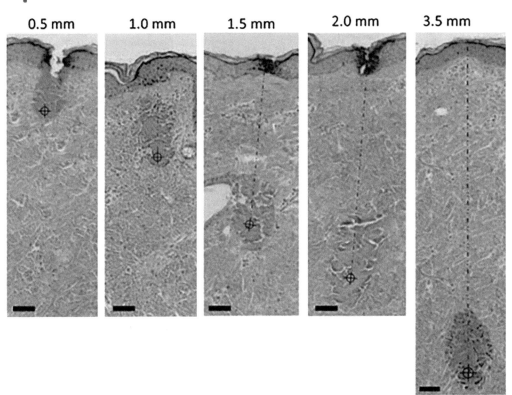

Fig. 2. Columns of coagulation created by an insulated RFM device with a variable-depth tip. (*Courtesy of* Medical and Science Affairs, Lutronic Corporation, Gyeonggi-do, South Korea.)

and new collagen deposition.[22] This is the process of collagen denaturing and is seen in conjunction with the coagulation process noted above (**Box 1**).

INSULATED VERSUS NONINSULATED NEEDLES

Insulated needles theoretically allow for RF energy placement into the dermis while protecting the epidermis from most of the heat. There will always be some heat transmitted superficially from the deeper layers just through proximity and conduction as the heat gradually dissipates. Also, there may be heat transferred through the insulation, particularly with more aggressive treatment settings. Energy can transmit superficially along the exterior of the protected needle, although this was not seen in the preliminary studies of 1 of the RFM devices when the energy was delivered in a gel. Lastly, after several pulses, it is possible there is breakdown of the insulation, although this has never been studied.

Noninsulated needles will deliver a larger RTZ throughout the entire length of the electrode. Larger coagulation zones, despite being fractional, will heal slower than multiple small RTZs. Epidermal injuries may occur with the unprotected needles, thus leading to higher risks in darker skin types. In addition, wound care and downtime are potentially prolonged as these superficial wounds heal. With insulated needles, the epidermal injuries are limited to mechanical penetrations similar to simple microneedling and behave similar to these procedures with healing within 24 hours.

VARIABLE VERSUS FIXED-LENGTH NEEDLES

Variable lengths allow for more flexibility by the operator to treat different conditions and skin thickness. Even throughout the face, skin depths vary from 0.37 mm (eyelids) to over 2 mm. Acne scars and hyperhidrosis require deeper treatments, as deep as 2.5 to 3.5 mm in some cases. The fixed-length devices can work around this inherent problem by offering more than 1 tip, which adds additional costs.

Although dialing in a depth sounds eloquent, the exact location of the RTZ is not likely to lie precisely at the depth chosen (**Box 2**).

If the operator does not hold the handpiece perpendicular to the skin or without enough pressure, more superficial than desired RTZs will result. "Kickback" from the skin resistance is another reason for inexact RTZ placement. Thicker/scarred skin, dull needles (from poor manufacturing quality control or from multiple pulses), underpowered motor/solenoid can all lead to more shallow than anticipated depths. The more needles there are, the more resistance there is to penetration and the less likely the RTZs will be at the expected level. It must be kept in mind that there will be surrounding heating and coagulation of the exposed tips. Deeper heating is possible, but, most likely, more superficial than expected RTZs will occur. Note that the high impedance of the fat in the subcutaneous tissue is somewhat resistant to the heat from RF.

MANUAL VERSUS MECHANICAL INSERTION

With mechanical insertion, user variability should be reduced. Unfortunately, many systems have underpowered motors/solenoids, which are unable to overcome the inherent resistance of the skin to get to their desired depths. With manual insertion devices, there is operator fatigue, which will factor into the equation, particularly when there are multiple treatments in 1 day or multiple areas are treated on the same patient.

Some systems rely on the manual insertion of fixed-length pins/needles. The completion of the electric current requires the handpiece to be flush with the patient's skin because the return electrode rests on the immediate adjacent skin. With

---

Box 1
Variations among radiofrequency microneedling devices

- Insulated versus noninsulated needles
- Variable versus length needles
- Manual versus mechanical insertion
- Bipolar versus monopolar
- Temperature/impedance feedback versus none
- Pulse durations
- Bulk versus fractional heating
- Motor versus solenoid insertion

Box 2
Variables preventing precise placement

- Technique of operator
- Depth chosen
- Characteristics/resistance of tissues
- Needle sharpness
- Number of needles
- Power of motor/solenoid

the rapidity of the treatment, there is bound to be some "imperfect" pulses leading to arcing across the epidermis with a resultant burn because of inexact handpiece seating or fluid/blood of skin surface. In addition, these devices and the other uninsulated needle devices produce superficial ablative injuries in the epidermis, creating a scarring risk and additional downtime. If the energy flow is analyzed, there is both bulk and fractional heating with these devices, which can create more downtime and risk versus a true fractional RTZ.

TEMPERATURE AND IMPEDANCE FEEDBACK

Radiofrequency energy transmission is highly dependent of the hydration of the skin, collagen, and electrolyte content, and many other variables (see later discussion). It has also been established that there is a threshold that is needed (65°C–70°C) to obtain coagulation and maximal neocollagenesis. One device monitors temperature and impedance, which gives instantaneous feedback to the handpiece to maintain the temperature at 67°C during its 3- to 5-second pulse. We also know that too much current causes desiccation and termination of energy flow. Another device monitors impedance and, through a feedback loop, delivers a specified amount of energy during the pulse. Unfortunately, most of the RFM devices use no tissue monitoring and results are not optimized (**Table 1**).

TREATMENT PROTOCOLS

On the day of treatment, informed consent and photographs are taken. Photos, with and without flash, should be obtained from both sides of the face, at 0°, 45°, and 90°, with and without expression. For further documentation, 3D photos should be taken, if available. The treated area should be cleansed, and topical anesthetic should be applied. Typically, a compounded mixture of beta-caine, lidocaine, and tetracaine is commonly used, but offices have their preferences for a variety of topical anesthetics. After the appropriate time period, the cream/ointment is removed, and the face is again cleaned and sterilized. Rubbing alcohol, chlorhexidine, and hypochlorous acid are the preferred ways to prep the face before treatment. It is essential that sterility be maintained during the procedure because there is a significant disruption of the skin's epidermal barrier for the next 12 to 24 hours. Postprocedure acne flairs are often superficial infections related to lapses in sterile technique. In addition, application of topical clindamycin or hypochlorous acid or preventative oral antibiotics will cut down on the incidence of acne significantly.

PROCEDURE DISCOMFORT

Probably the primary complaint with regard to RFM procedures is pain. There are many measures, as outlined previously, to make the treatment more comfortable. Pulse duration seems to directly correlate to discomfort,[9] and is why a device with long 2- to 4-second pulses requires tumescent anesthesia. It is promoted as a "1 and done" procedure, so patients will often opt for this despite more downtime (large RTZs) and the required tumescence. Many other RFM devices cause little to no pain after topical anesthesia. Careful observation will show whether the penetration of the microneedles is poor and energy delivery is low. In the author's opinion, the efficacy of "painless" RFM devices must be questioned. Energy delivery into the mid-dermis is inherently painful (**Box 3**).

Procedure time varies according to the device and varies from about 15 to 60 minutes. Bleeding is usually minimal and should be wiped with sterile gauze, which is particularly important when the surface electrode completes the circuit, as is true of a few devices. Taking breaks to allow the patient to "regroup" is sometimes necessary, but should not prolong the procedure too long (**Box 4**).

TREATMENT PARAMETERS

Inherently, higher-energy treatments should yield better results. Studies have shown that the amount of collagen produced is directly dependent on the intensity of heating of the connective tissue.[10,23–25] In a study by Hruza and colleagues,[26] higher-energy treatments yielded better clinical results. In contrast, a 5-person study (performed by the author) in which 7–8 J/pulse was given, the patient results were deemed similar to patients treated with 3–5 J/pulse, but the downtime was extended to 3 to 4 weeks (redness, grid marks). This downtime was unacceptable in the author's opinion and was contradictory to the attractiveness of minimal downtime RF procedures. In a similar study using fractional bipolar RF comparing higher versus moderate energy levels, there were more side effects with the higher settings, but comparable results at 3 and 6 month follow-up.[27] It seems like there is a plateau in which higher energies give no additional benefit, but add to downtime and side effects.

In studies with 1 particular RFM device, high treatment levels (TLs) with short pulse durations led to spikes in the impedance, which terminated

Table 1
Current radiofrequency microneedling devices

Device	Company	Needle Depth (mm)	No. of Needles	Insulated/Noninsulated	Fractional/Bulk	Motorized/Manual	Unique Characteristics
Infini	Lutronic	0.25–3.5	49	Insulated	Fractional	Motorized	High-energy painful; sounds like stapler
Intensif	Endymed	0.5–5.0	25	Noninsulated	Fractional	Motorized	Max pulse duration 200 ms limits energy; noninsulated risks PIH
Profound	Syneron Candela	5 (at 25° and 75°)	10	Insulated	Fractional	Manual	Pulse 3–5 s, painful; temperature feedback; skin quality tip for cellulite
Secret	Cutera	0.5–3.5	25/64	Noninsulated/Insulated	Fractional	Motorized	Offers insulated and noninsulated tips
Fractora	Inmode	Multiple tips up to 3	24/60/126	Noninsulated/Insulated	Fractional and bulk	Manual	Energy flow risks epidermis—blister/PIH; fixed needle depths
eMatrix	Syneron Candela	0.5	44/64	Noninsulated	Fractional and bulk	Manual	Energy flow risks epidermis—blister/PIH; fixed needle depths
Vivace	Aesthetics Biomedical	0.5–3.5	36	Insulated	Fractional	Motorized	Motor underpowered?
Intracel	Jeisys Perigee	0.1–2.0	36	Insulated	Fractional	Motorized	Has monopolar mode to get deeper penetration
Genius	Lutronic	0.5–4.5	49	Insulated	Fractional	Motorized	Impedance feedback to optimize energy; fewer side effects
Voluderm	Lumenis	0.6/1.0	24/36	Noninsulated	Fractional	Manual	RF during entire pulse eases insertion; PIH risk
Viva	Venus Concept	0.5	160	Noninsulated	Fractional	Motorized	SmartScan changes energy density without changing tip; resurfaces
Morpheus8	Inmode	2–4/8	25	Insulated	Fractional	Motorized	Able to destroy fat with up to 8 mm depths

Box 3
Measures to assist in patient comfort when topical anesthetics do not fully accommodate a pain-free treatment

- Nerve blocks
- Superficial skin injections with anesthetic—"superficial skin block" with a multiple-needle injector
- Tumescent anesthesia
- Oral narcotics or antianxiolytics
- Nitrous oxide/oxygen mixture—fixed 50%/50% ratio
- Cold air/cold devices/ice—forced air coolers
- Vibration—gate theory
- "Talkasthesia"
- Music (room or headphones)

Box 4
Techniques to minimize risks/downtime/complications

- Always keep the handpiece perpendicular in all directions to the skin
- Maintain firm pressure on the handpiece to ensure appropriate depth of the needles
- Avoid stacking pulses
- Allow for skin cooling—alternate sides if multiple passes/small areas require breaks before additional passes
- Choose appropriate power settings and depths for the skin condition/area of body or face/skin type
- Maintain sterility throughout procedure
- Avoid superficial depths in Fitzpatrick skin type IV-VI
- Higher energies should be reserved for deeper passes only

Box 5
Other instructions given to the patient

- Avoid all make up application until the following day
- Apply the recommended topicals (healing gels, growth factor serums similar to postablative laser)
- Sun exposure—best practice is not established; safer to avoid sun
- Exercise–no restrictions
- Elevate the head of treat area with several pillows to decrease edema for 2 days
- Cleanse the skin before sleeping and in the morning with gentle cleanser

Box 6
Short-term complications

- Bruising, petechia
- Acne flair
- Superficial infection
- Persistent "grid/track" marks
- Redness and edema
- Superficial burn
- Postinflammatory hyperpigmentation

the RF pulses prematurely. Histologically, this phenomenon was attributed to tissue desiccation surrounding the RTZs. The RF energy could not propagate through the tissue depleted of water. There are certain devices with temperature or impedance measurement built into the needles to give feedback, with adjustments of the energy output performed automatically. The devices with feedback will give a more definitive and consistent delivery on energy than one without this feature because there are numerous variables affecting impedance (as previously stated). Studies performed by the author using one particular device have shown that optimal energy delivery was obtained using lower TLs with longer pulse durations (300–500 ms) rather than short pulses with higher TLs. Second and third passes transmit higher energies because the heat from pervious passes lowers the impedance of the tissue.[22]

Another consideration for choosing energy parameters is the size of the resultant RTZs. During the healing process, replacement of the RTZs with newly formed collagen, there will be faster repair with smaller RTZs because of the higher surface area to volume ratio. There will be longer downtimes with larger RTZs and more risk if the pulse is not placed perfectly. The Profound

Box 7
RFM is currently being used for multiple indications

- Aging—wrinkles and tightening
- Acne scars
- Acne
- Axillary hyperhidrosis
- Cellulite
- Striae—stretch marks
- Hair thinning/alopecia
- Rosacea/postinflammatory erythema

Table 2
Table of studies

Indication	Author(s), Year	No. of Patients In Study	Purpose	Findings of Study/ Paper
Antiaging	Alexiades-Armenakas et al,[37] 2010	25	Compare RFM with facelift	RFM improved skin laxity 37% of facelift with less risk
Antiaging	Alexiades-Armenakas et al,[38] 2013	100	Neck and face laxity/wrinkles	100% improved, average 25% wrinkle reduction; 66.7°C, 4.2 s optimal; 90% satisfied
Antiaging	Calderhead et al,[39] 2013	499	Safety and wrinkles	80%–88% satisfaction, minimal adverse effects (AE), types I-V
Periorbital rytids	Kim et al,[40] 2013	11	Periobital wrinkles	10/11 very satisfied after 3 treatments; minimum downtime/side effects
Antiaging	Hruza et al,[26] 2009	35	Skin quality and wrinkles	80%–90% had improvement in skin brightness, tightness, smoothness
Neck	Clementoni & Munavalli,[34] 2016	33	Neck tightness	Decreased cervicomental and gnathion angles of 28.58° and 16.68°
Acne scars	Park et al,[31] 2016	20	Acne scars	All had grade 2 improvement in scars or greater
Acne scars	Chandrashekar et al,[33] 2014	31	Acne scars skin types 3–5	80% grade 2, 20% grade 1 improvement; PIH 5 track marks 2
Acne scars	Oblepias,[41] 2010	20	Acne scars	72% had great or very great improvement
Axillary hyperhidrosis	Kim et al,[42] 2013	20	Hyperhidrosis	Hyperhidrosis Disease Severity Scale (HDSS) scores 3.5 baseline to 2.3 after 8 wk
Axillary hyperhidrosis	Naeini et al,[43] 2015	25	Sham control study	79% decreased HDSS scores by 1%–2%, 80% had 50% satisfaction or higher
Cellulite	Alexiades et al,[44] 2018	50	Cellulite	93% success rate at 6 mo
Abdominal striae	Harmelin et al,[45] 2016	22	Bipolar RF plus RFM/Light	21.6% decrease in depth, no change in width

(continued on next page)

Table 2
(continued)

Indication	Author(s), Year	No. of Patients In Study	Purpose	Findings of Study/ Paper
Abdominal striae	Naeini et al,[46] 2016	6	RFM with/without CO_2	Better with CO_2
Acne vulgaris	Lee et al,[47] 2012	18	Acne control	All had grade 2–4 improvement, none worsened
Hair loss	Yu et al,[48] 2018	19	Minoxidil with/ without RFM	Higher hair count and thickness on RFM side of scalp
Postinflammatory erythema	Min et al,[49] 2015	25	Erythema	Effective for postinflammatory erythema; anti-inflammatory and antiangiogenic effects
Acne vulgaris	Lee et al,[50] 2013	20	Sebum production	Sebum decreased for 8 wk and returned after 1 treatment
Acne scars	Faghihi et al,[51] 2017	25	RFM with/without subcision	Subcision + RFM better
Acne scars and pores	Cho et al,[52] 2012	30	Large pores and acne scars	70% or more improvement in large pores and acne scars all patients
Acne vulgaris	Kwon et al,[53] 2018	25	Compare RFM with laser split face	RFM more prolonged results
Acne and acne scars	Min et al,[54] 2015	20	Compare RFM vs bipolar (epidermal) RF	RFM superior to bipolar (epidermal) RF
Acne vulgaris	Kim et al,[55] 2014	25	Acne reduction	78% acne reduction, 37% sebum reduction
Safety	Cohen et al,[35] 2016	30	Safety with insulated needles	Minimal downtime and no AE
Acne scars/safety	Ibrahimi et al,[36] 2015	4	Safety in acne scars/dark skin	Safe without AE
Axillary hyperhidrosis	Abtahi-Naeini et al,[56] 2016	25	Long-term effectiveness	45.9% relapse after 1 y. Higher body mass index, more relapse
Axillary hyperhidrosis	Chilukuri et al,[57] 2018	N/A	Efficacy of RFM	Beneficial for long-term control of sweating

produces the largest RTZs and is claimed to have a 30% dermal coverage with its "1and done" treatments.

ADJUNCTIVE TREATMENTS

The RFM procedures are often done in combination with other procedures and have proven to be safe in this regard. Skin resurfacing with ablative and nonablative lasers can target the epidermis—pigmentation, scarring, fine lines—which are not addressed with most of the RFM devices. To address acne scarring/volume deficits, chemical reconstruction of skin scars using trichloroacetic acid, dermal fillers, subcision, and platelet-rich plasma (PRP) have been performed on the same day by the author without any increased side effects or risks. In a 2017 study by Dr. Lim, various hyaluronic acid and calcium hydroxyapatite fillers were injected into a test subject's back. After treating the areas with RFM, biopsies were taken to access the effect on the fillers. Findings showed that there was no effect on the fillers at all energies levels. PRP (high concentration 5–9×) seems to help speed up the healing process. Studies have shown better results for acne scars when PRP is used in conjunction with microneedling than microneedling alone. Postprocedure use of light-emitting diodes-low laser light at 830 nm seems to calm the skin, improves healing times, and improves outcomes.[28]

POSTPROCEDURE CARE

The microneedle channels stay patent for varying durations, dependent on the size of needles, depth, and energies, but it is estimated to be for 6 to 12 hours. It is imperative that the patient maintain a clean environment around the treat area for at least this amount of time. There are cases of granuloma formation following microneedling procedures with topical therapies,[29] so caution is needed when choosing the appropriate creams/serums (**Box 5**).

SAFETY AND COMPLICATIONS

In general, the RFM procedure is extremely safe with minimal downtime.[8,10,11,18,30–36] The expected postprocedure recovery consists of erythema, edema, and minor skin flaking for about 2 to 3 days. With higher-energy devices or settings, this can be extended to up to 1 week (**Box 6**).

These will all improve with observation or appropriate therapy. Long-term complications are extremely rare—scarring and skin textural abnormalities. It must be emphasized that provider technique is most likely the cause of complications because RFM devices are inherently safe (**Box 7**).

The therapeutic benefits of RFM has been thoroughly examined and documented with multiple studies (**Table 2**). As seen in the table, skin laxity, brightness, and smoothness (wrinkles) have all shown improvement because of the collagen remodeling/formation and neoelastinogenesis from RFM. Acne scarring treatments have been revolutionized with RFM because of the increased depths, reverse thermal gradient, and minimal epidermal thermal injury (particularly important in the darker skin types). Permanent control of hyperhidrosis with 1 to 3 treatments has been achieved with histologically confirmed destruction of sweat glands, although a study by Naeini and

colleagues[43] suggested relapse in 1 year in 46% of patients. Cellulite treatment showed improvement in the study by Alexiades. Stretch marks showed improvement when used in combination with lasers but width was unchanged. A split head study showed RFM was beneficial in combination with minoxidil versus minoxidil alone. Improvement in controlling redness related to rosacea and postinflammatory erythema has also been shown with RFM.

SUMMARY

RFM is a significant advance over traditional RF devices for skin tightening with improvements in safety and efficacy. Energy delivery is efficient into the dermis with minimal disruption of the epidermis, particularly for the insulated needle devices. The devices that monitor tissue characteristics (temperature and impedance) should optimize patient outcomes and safety. RFM should be considered the new standard for treating acne scarring, particularly in darker skin types, as well as the minimal invasive neck rejuvenation/laxity solution.

REFERENCES

1. Sadick NS, Makino Y. Selective electro-thermolysis in aesthetic medicine: a review. Lasers Surg Med 2004;34:91–7.
2. Belenky I, Margulis A, Elman M, et al. Exploring channeling optimized radiofrequency energy: a review of radiofrequency history and applications in esthetic fields. Adv Ther 2012;29(3):249–66.
3. Gold MH. The increasing use of nonablative radiofrequency in the rejuvenation of the skin. Expert Rev Dermatol 2011;6(2):139–43.
4. Schepps JL, Foster KR. The UHF and microwave dielectric properties of normal and tumour tissues: variation in dielectric properties with tissue water content. Phys Med Biol 1980;25:1149–59.
5. Beasley KL, Weiss RA. Radiofrequency in cosmetic dermatology. Dermatol Clin 2014;32:79–90.
6. De Felipe I, Del Cueto SR, Perez E, et al. Adverse reactions after nonablative radiofrequency: follow-up of 290 patients. J Cosmet Dermatol 2007;6(3): 163–6.
7. Alster TS, Lupton JR. Nonablative cutaneous remodeling using radiofrequency devices. Clin Dermatol 2007;25:487–91.
8. Clementoni MT, Munavalli GS. Fractional high intensity focused radiofrequency in the treatment of mild to moderate laxity of the lower face and neck: a pilot study. Lasers Surg Med 2016;48(5):461–70.
9. Hayashi K, Thabit G, Massa KL, et al. The effect of thermal heating on the length and histologic

properties of the glenohumeral joint capsule. Am J Sports Med 1997;25:107–12.

10. Yeo L, Lim – Presented at ASLMS Annual Meeting 2010, Phoenix, Arizona.

11. Abraham MT, Vic Ross E. Current concepts in nonablative radiofrequency rejuvenation of the lower face and neck. Facial Plast Surg 2005;21(1):65–73.

12. Bernstein LJ, Kauvar AN, Grossman MC, et al. The short- and long-term side effects of carbon dioxide laser resurfacing. Dermatol Surg 1997;23(7):519–25.

13. Preissig J, Hamilton K, Markus R. Current laser resurfacing technolgies: a review that delves beneath the surface. Semin Plast Surg 2012;26(3):109–16.

14. Chan HHL, Manstein D, Yu CS, et al. The prevalence and risk factors of post inflammatory hyperpigmentation after fractional resurfacing in Asians. Lasers Surg Med 2007;39(5):381–5.

15. Chwalek J, Goldberg DJ. Ablative skin resurfacing. Curr Probl Dermatol 2011;42:40–7.

16. Fife DJ, Fitzpatrick RE, Zachary CB. Complications of fractional CO_2 laser resurfacing: four cases. Lasers Surg Med 2009;41(3):179–84.

17. Avram MM, Tope WD, MPhil M, et al. Hypertrophic scarring of the neck following ablative fractional carbon dioxide laser resurfacing. Lasers Surg Med 2009;41(3):185–8.

18. Hantash BM, Renton B, Berkowitz RL, et al. Pilot clinical study of a novel minimally invasive bipolar microneedle radiofrequency device. Lasers Surg Med 2009;41(2):87–95.

19. Hantash BM, Ubeid AA, Chang H, et al. Bipolar fractional radiofrequency treatment induces neoelastogenesis and neocollagenesis. Lasers Surg Med 2009;41(1):1–9.

20. Zheng Z, Goo B, Kim DY, et al. Histometric analysis of skin-radiofrequency interaction using a fractionated microneedle delivery system. Dermatol Surg 2014;40:134–41.

21. Thomsen S. Pathologic analysis of photothermal and photomechanical effects of laser-tissue interactions. Photochem Photobiol 1991;53:825–35.

22. Sadick N. Tissue tightening technologies: fact or fiction. Aesthet Surg J 2008;28:180–8.

23. Zelickson BD, Kist D, Bernstein E, et al. Histological and ultrastructural evaluation of the effects of a radiofrequency-based nonablative dermal remodeling device. Arch Dermatol 2004;140:204–9.

24. Kuo T, Speyer MT, Ries WR, et al. Collagen thermal damage and collagen synthesis after cutaneous laser resurfacing. Lasers Surg Med 1998;23:66–71.

25. Goldberg DJ. Nonablative dermal remodeling: does it really work? Arch Dermatol 2002;138:1366–8.

26. Hruza G, Taub AF, Collier SL, et al. Skin rejuvenation and wrinkle reduction using a fractional radiofrequency system. J Drugs Dermatol 2009;8(3):259–65.

27. Phothong W, Wanitphakdeedecha R, Sathaworawong A, et al. High versus moderate energy use of bipolar fractional radiofrequency in the treatment of acne scars: a split-face double-blinded randomized control trial pilot study. Lasers Med Sci 2016;31(2):229–34.

28. Calderhead G. Combining microneedle fractional radiofrequency and LED photoactivation. Prime 2014;2(6):15–23.

29. Soltani-Arabshahi R, Wong JW, Duffy KL, et al. Facial allergic granulomatosis reaction and systemic hypersensitivity associated with microneedle therapy for skin rejuvenation. JAMA Dermatol 2014;150(1):68–72.

30. Martin J. Review of fractional microneedling radiofrequency for skin rejuvenation. Prime 2018;6(3).

31. Park JY, Lee EG, Yoon MS, et al. The efficacy and safety of combined microneedle fractional radiofrequency and sublative fractional radiofrequency for acne scars in Asian skin. J Cosmet Dermatol 2016;15(2):102–7.

32. Cohen JL, Weiner SF, Pozner JN, et al. Multi-center pilot study to evaluate the safety profile of high energy fractionated radiofrequency with insulated microneedles to multiple levels of the dermis. J Drugs Dermatol 2016;15(11):1308–12.

33. Chandrashekar BS, Sriram R, Mysore R, et al. Evaluation of microneedling fractional radiofrequency device for treatment of acne scars. J Cutan Aesthet Surg 2014;7(2):93–7.

34. Clementoni MT, Munavalli GS. Fractional high intensity focused radiofrequency in the treatment of mild to moderate laxity of the lower face and neck: a pilot study. Lasers Surg Med 2016;48(5):461–70.

35. Cohen JL, Weiner SF, Pozner JN, et al. Multi-Center Pilot Study to evaluate the safety profile of high energy fractionated radiofrequency with insulated microneedles to multiple levels of the dermis. J Drugs Dermatol 2016;15(11):1308–12.

36. Ibrahimi OA, Weiss RA, Weiss MA, et al. Treatment of acne scars with high intensity focused radio frequency. J Drugs Dermatol 2015;14(9):1065–8.

37. Alexiades-Armenakas M, Rosenberg D, Renton B, et al. Blinded, randomized, quantitative grading comparison of minimally invasive, fractional radiofrequency and surgical face-lift to treat skin laxity. Arch Dermatol 2010;146(4):396–405.

38. Alexiades-Armenakas M, Newman J, Willey A, et al. Prospective multicenter clinical trial of a minimally invasive temperature-controlled bipolar fractional radiofrequency system for rhytid and laxity treatment. Dermatol Surg 2013;39(2):263–73.

39. Calderhead RG, Goo BL, Lauro F, et al. The clinical efficacy and safety of microneedling fractional radiofrequency in the treatment of facial wrinkles: a multicenter study with the INFINI system in 499 patients. 2013. Available at: www.lutronic.com.

40. Kim JK, Roh MR, Park GH, et al. Fractionated micro-needle radiofrequency for the treatment of periorbital wrinkles. J Dermatol 2013;40(3):172–6.

41. Oblepias MSM. Open label study on the safety and efficacy of radiofrequency with microneedle (Intracel) on mild to severe acne scars in Asian skin. International master course on aging skin, Asia 2010. Available at: https://perigee.com/wp-content/uploads/INTRAcel-Jeisys-Article.pdf.

42. Kim M, Shin JY, Lee J, et al. Efficacy of fractional microneedle radiofrequency device in the treatment of primary axillary hyperhidrosis: a pilot study. Dermatology 2013;227:243–9.

43. Naeini F, Abtahi-Naeini B, Pourazizi M, et al. Fractionated microneedle radiofrequency for treatment of primary axillary hyperhidrosis: a sham control study. Australas J Dermatol 2015. https://doi.org/10.1111/ajd.12260.

44. Alexiades M, Munavalli G, Goldberg D, et al. Prospective multicenter clinical trial of a temperature-controlled subcutaneous microneedle fractional bipolar radiofrequency system for the treatment of cellulite. Dermatol Surg 2018;44(10):1262–71.

45. Harmelin Y, Boineau D, Cardot-Leccia N, et al. Fractionated bipolar radiofrequency and bipolar radiofrequency potentiated by infrared light for treating striae: a prospective randomized, comparative trial with objective evaluation. Lasers Surg Med 2016;48(3):245–53.

46. Naeini FF, Behfar S, Abtahi-Naeini B, et al. Promising option for treatment of striae alba: fractionated microneedle radiofrequency in combination with fractional carbon dioxide laser. Dermatol Res Pract 2016;2016:2896345.

47. Lee SJ, Goo JW, Shin J, et al. Use of fractionated microneedle radiofrequency for the treatment of inflammatory acne vulgaris in 18 Korean patients. Dermatol Surg 2012;38(3):400–5.

48. Yu AJ, Luo YJ, Xu XG, et al. A pilot split-scalp study of combined fractional radiofrequency microneedling and 5% topical minoxidil in treating male pattern hair loss. Clin Exp Dermatol 2018;43(7):775–81.

49. Min S, Park SY, Yoon JY, et al. Fractional microneedling radiofrequency treatment for acne-related post-inflammatory erythema. Acta Derm Venereol 2015;96(1):87–91.

50. Lee KR, Lee EG, Lee HJ, et al. Assessment of treatment efficacy and sebosuppressive effect of fractional radiofrequency microneedle on acne vulgaris. Lasers Surg Med 2013;45(10):639–47.

51. Faghihi G, Poostiyan N, Asilian A, et al. Efficacy of fractionated microneedle radiofrequency with and without adding subcision for the treatment of atrophic facial acne scars: a randomized split-face clinical study. J Cosmet Dermatol 2017;16(Suppl 2):223–9.

52. Cho SI, Chung BY, Choi MG, et al. Evaluation of the clinical efficacy of fractional radiofrequency microneedle treatment in acne scars and large facial pores. Dermatol Surg 2012;38(7 Pt 1):1017–24.

53. Kwon HH, Park HY, Choi SC, et al. Novel device-based acne treatments: comparison of a 1450-nm diode laser and microneedling radiofrequency on mild-to-moderate acne vulgaris and seborrhoea in Korean patients through a 20-week prospective, randomized, split-face study. J Eur Acad Dermatol Venereol 2018;32(4):639–44.

54. Min S, Park SY, Yoon JY, et al. Comparison of fractional microneedling radiofrequency and bipolar radiofrequency on acne and acne scar and investigation of mechanism: comparative randomized controlled clinical trial. Arch Dermatol Res 2015;307(10):897–904.

55. Kim ST, Lee KH, Sim HJ, et al. Treatment of acne vulgaris with fractional radiofrequency microneedling. J Dermatol 2014;41(7):586–91.

56. Abtahi-Naeini B, Naeini FF, Saffaei A, et al. Treatment of primary axillary hyperhidrosis by fractional microneedle radiofrequency: is it still effective after long-term follow-up? Indian J Dermatol 2016;61(2):234.

57. Chilukuri S, Robb CW, Weiner SF, et al. Primary axillary hyperhidrosis treatment using high intensity focused fractional radiofrequency microneedling. J Drugs Dermatol 2018;17(7):745–8.

Percutaneous Radiofrequency Technologies for the Lower Face and Neck

Garrett D. Locketz, MD[a], Jason D. Bloom, MD[a,b],*

KEYWORDS

- Radiofrequency • Percutaneous • Subdermal • Cervical rejuvenation • ThermiTight • FaceTite
- Inmode • Thermi

KEY POINTS

- The neck contour contributes significantly to overall facial aesthetics; the aging neck frequently displays subcutaneous and subplatysmal fat, which blunts the cervicomental angle.
- Stigma of surgery, fear of morbidity, and increased time in the public eye has led patients to desire less invasive treatments, earlier in life, with less morbidity and downtime.
- Percutaneous radiofrequency technologies safely and effectively ablate subcutaneous fat and tighten skin by delivering energy directly into the subdermal space.
- In select patients, percutaneous radiofrequency treatment yields a 30% to 40% contraction at 6 months and 40% to 50% at 1 year.
- Percutaneous radiofrequency treatment is a one-time, no sutures, no scalpels, no surgery procedure performed in the office under local anesthesia with long-lasting effects and minimal downtime.

 Video content accompanies this article at http://www.facialplastic.theclinics.com.

INTRODUCTION

In aesthetic medicine, the gold standard for treatment of skin laxity is surgical excision. Yet in recent years, stigma of surgery, fear of morbidity, and increased time in the public eye via social media has led many patients to desire less invasive treatments, earlier in life, with less morbidity and downtime. With respect to facial aesthetics, the neck subunit often ages earlier and more noticeably than others and is one of the most common motivations for patients to present for rejuvenation options.

Controlled disruption and subsequent remodeling of dermal and subdermal collagen is the underlying mechanism of nonsurgical skin rejuvenation. In the neck, the hypodermis contains a complex collagen network involving the papillary and reticular dermis, fibroseptal network intermixed with subcutaneous fat, and underlying fibrous fascia. These deeper tissue layers act in concert with the more superficial dermal skin layers to create the skin's tone, quality, and durability. In addition to ptotic skin, the aging neck frequently displays subcutaneous and subplatysmal fat, which blunts the cervicomental angle and contributes to an

Disclosure Statement: Dr J.D. Bloom is an advisor/consultant to and on the speaker's bureau to both ThermiAesthetics and InMode and Dr G.D. Locketz has nothing to disclose.
[a] Department of Otolaryngology–Head & Neck Surgery, Division of Facial Plastic Surgery, University of Pennsylvania, 3400 Spruce Street, Philadelphia, PA 19146, USA; [b] Main Line Center for Laser Surgery, 32 Parking Plaza, Suite 200, Ardmore, PA 19003, USA
* Corresponding author. 32 Parking Plaza, Suite 200, Ardmore, PA 19003.
E-mail address: drjbloom@hotmail.com

Facial Plast Surg Clin N Am 27 (2019) 305–320
https://doi.org/10.1016/j.fsc.2019.03.003
1064-7406/19/© 2019 Elsevier Inc. All rights reserved.

aged aesthetic. Traditionally, noninvasive cervical rejuvenation has been accomplished via chemical ablation, light- or laser-based technologies, ultrasonic energy, or transcutaneous radiofrequency (RF) devices. Although each of these technologies has their indications and merits, their results are either modest skin tightening requiring multiple procedures that often fail to meet patients' expectations, or significant skin tightening at the risk of excessive morbidity. These technologies also fail to address subdermal adipose tissue, which limits their effectiveness in many patients presenting for rejuvenation. Liposuction has been used for many years in the minimally invasive setting to remove submental fat; however, many patients presenting for neck rejuvenation have poor skin tone that fails to recoil and fill the dead space after fat removal, resulting in an overall unfavorable aesthetic outcome.

Recently, percutaneous RF technologies have been introduced to simultaneously ablate subcutaneous fat and tighten the overlying skin.[1–5] These technologies safely and effectively apply energy directly into the subdermal space, targeting the upper dermal collagen network, the deeper fascial layer, and fibrofatty septum, which anchors the dermis to the deep fascia. Significant skin tightening and fat reduction have been reported with these technologies, beyond that which is currently achievable with other minimally invasive energy-based technologies.

This article focuses on percutaneous, subdermal RF devices, highlighting the physiology of skin tightening, the overall energy-based skin tightening landscape that led to the development of these technologies, the procedural steps to using these technologies, and a discussion of their indications and results.

GENERAL STATISTICS

In the annual Plastic Surgery Statistics report published by the American Society of Plastic Surgery, 1.8 million surgical cosmetic procedures and 15.7 million minimally invasive cosmetic procedures were performed in 2017. Among the surgical procedures, liposuction (including treatments to body and neck) ranked number 2 at nearly 250,000 treatments, a 5% increase from the previous year. Facial and neck rejuvenation accounted for the majority of minimally invasive procedures, with 2 of the 5 most popular treatments being procedures aimed skin tightening (chemical peel and microdermabrasion), combining for 2.1 million treatments performed.[6] This trend of increasing demand for minimally invasive skin tightening and fat reduction is also evident in the dermatologic surgery domain.

According to the 2018 American Society for Dermatology Surgery consumer survey on cosmetic and dermatologic procedures, 70% of 3252 respondents reported considering various aesthetic procedures, up from 52% in 2014. Seventy-three percent of respondents were concerned by excess fat under the chin and neck, and the same percentage with skin texture, discoloration, or both. Fifty-seven percent of respondents were considering procedures to tighten skin or smooth wrinkles using ultrasound, laser, light, or RF treatments.[7]

ANATOMY

The contour of the neck contributes significantly to overall facial aesthetics. A youthful neck is characterized by an acute cervicomental angle with a firm and well-defined jawline. The skin is smooth without dyschromia, rhytids, or platysmal banding. Submandibular glands are tightly bound beneath the mandibular border, and jowling is absent anteriorly (**Fig. 1**). In contrast, the aged/aging neck is characterized by submental adiposity with blunting of the cervicomental angle, platysmal banding, and ptotic dyspigmented skin with vertical and horizontal rhytids. The epidermis is thickened, there is an accumulation of elastotic collagen whorls, decreased dermal thickness, and in many cases, subplatysmal fat accompanies subdermal adiposity (**Fig. 2**).[8]

Youthful Neck

- Acute cervicomental angle[8]
- A firm, well-defined jawline
- Skin is smooth and devoid of horizontal or vertical neck lines
- Smooth and even platysma without banding
- Without visible submandibular glands or jowling
- Skin that is bright and even in color with minimal melanin or vascular lesions

Aging Neck

- Blunted, obtuse cervicomental angle[8]
- Poorly defined jawline with jowling
- Skin is rough with dyschromia and telangiectasia
- Thickened epidermis and decreased dermal thickness
- Decrease in collagen, elastin, and ground substances, with an accumulation of elastotic collage whorls in the deep dermis
- Atrophy of the platysma muscle with banding
- Accumulation of subplatysmal and subcutaneous fat in the submentum

- acute cervicomental angle
- defined jawline
- smooth, even, bright skin
- no horizontal or vertical lines
- no platysmal bands
- no visible submandibular glands
- non-hypertrophic masseter muscles
- Minimal melanin or vascular lesions

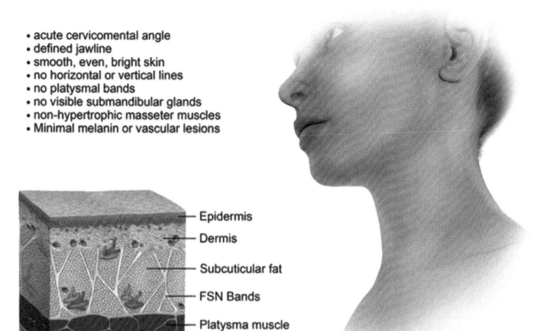

— Epidermis

— Dermis

— Subcuticular fat

— FSN Bands

— Platysma muscle

— Subplatysmal fat

Fig. 1. The ideal youthful neck. (*From* Mulholland RS. Nonexcisional, minimally invasive rejuvenation of the neck. Clin Plast Surg 2014;41(1):12; with permission.)

Cervical subcutaneous fat

A wide variation in the presentation of aging exists with respect to the cervical subcutaneous layer. Subcutaneous and supraplastysmal fat is found in the deep subdermis, superficial to the platysma muscle and is generally distributed between suprahyoid and infrahyoid compartments. Some patients with aging necks have little fat between the deep dermis and the platysma, whereas others display an extensive amount. Regardless, even modest amounts of subcutaneous cervical fat create an obtuse cervicomental angle and distract from a youthful appearance.

In conjunction with the increase in obesity worldwide, a variety of techniques have been developed over the past 30 years to treat submental and cervical adiposity. Conventional body liposuction is performed in the deep adipose layer, which limits the potential for postoperative contour deformities and dermal damage.[9] Superficial, subcutaneous liposuction was first described in the mid 1980s,[10] and, since then, numerous modifications, devices, and techniques have been developed.[9] Shortly after introduction, superficial suction-assisted liposuction (SAL) was adapted from body contouring for use in the neck to treat subcutaneous, preplatysmal adiposity.[8]

SAL is based on mechanical disruption of adipose tissue by suction. The cannula moves manually through the subcutaneous space and disrupts the adipose cells, while the suction aspirates small clusters of adipose through openings in the cannula.[3] Although the tumescent technique[11] developed in the late 1980s dramatically improved the postoperative recovery profile and safety, liposuction was still prone to significant postoperative edema, ecchymosis, and pain.

Documented skin contraction after SAL is minimal, ranging between the 6% and 10% at 1 year postoperatively, largely depending on the patient's inherent skin elasticity. Although this level of skin contraction can occasionally produce satisfactory results in select patients, the majority of patients with preplatysmal adiposity substantial enough to cause blunting of the cervicomental angle also have poor skin tone that will not contract and fill the dead space after SAL, resulting in an unfavorable cosmetic outcome. Furthermore, despite the multitude of advanced techniques and devices, SAL in the superficial subcutaneous fat plane is still prone to contour irregularities and skin ischemia.[9,12]

Energy based liposuction technologies were subsequently introduced, including ultrasound-assisted lipolysis and laser-assisted lipolysis

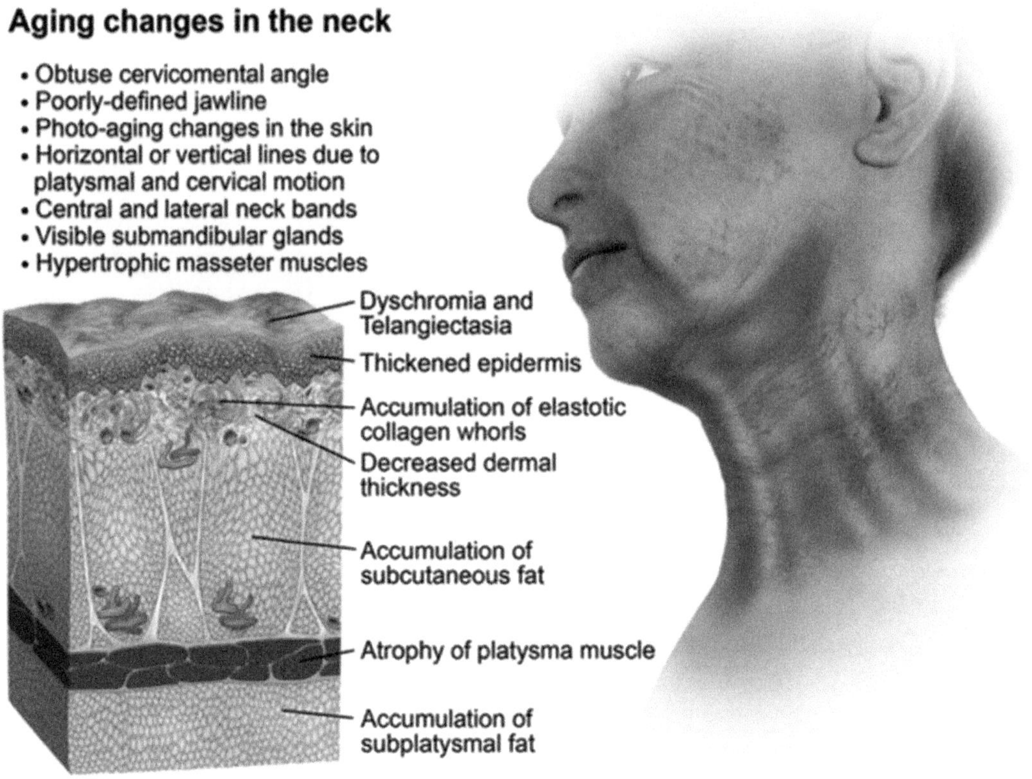

Aging changes in the neck

- Obtuse cervicomental angle
- Poorly-defined jawline
- Photo-aging changes in the skin
- Horizontal or vertical lines due to platysmal and cervical motion
- Central and lateral neck bands
- Visible submandibular glands
- Hypertrophic masseter muscles

Dyschromia and Telangiectasia

Thickened epidermis

Accumulation of elastotic collagen whorls

Decreased dermal thickness

Accumulation of subcutaneous fat

Atrophy of platysma muscle

Accumulation of subplatysmal fat

Fig. 2. The aging neck. (*From* Mulholland RS. Nonexcisional, minimally invasive rejuvenation of the neck. Clin Plast Surg 2014;41(1):13; with permission.)

(LAL), which resulted in less bleeding and bruising and enhanced recovery times versus SAL, although skin tightening was only modestly improved.[3,13–18]

CERVICAL SKIN TIGHTENING

The goal of all noninvasive skin tightening devices is to heat and remodel dermal and subcutaneous collagenous networks while avoiding collateral damage to unintended tissues.[19] Collagen consists of polymers held together by hydrogen bonds. The strength of collagen is directly proportional to the degree of hydrogen bond cross-linking.[20] Chemical or thermal energy delivered to collagen results in its denaturation, while the heat-stable intramolecular cross-links are preserved.[21] After this energy is applied, collagen fibrils ultimately undergo contraction and remodeling, which results in increased fibril size and strength.[2] Furthermore, thermal injury also results in the activation of wound-healing pathways, including recruitment of fibroblasts, which lay down new collagen leading to neocollagenesis[22]—whereby new collagen fills in surface

imperfections, resulting in more youthful appearing skin.[23]

Cervical Collagenous Network

- Dermis, both papillary and reticular
- Fascia, consisting of a thick layer of connective tissue located between the platysma and skin
- Fibrous septum (fibroseptal network or fibrofatty septum), consisting of thin layers of connective tissue separating lobules of fat and connecting the dermis with the fascia
- Reticular fibers, a framework of single collagen fibers encasing fat cells

By convention, the more ablative (or destructive) the technology, the greater potential for skin tightening. In older chemical ablation techniques, colloquially known as "chemical peels," topical agents applied to the skin created a chemical dissolution and coagulation of dermal proteins. The wound healing that followed over the next several weeks resulted in neocollagenesis, elastin production, and overall skin tightening.[8] Often, these techniques were difficult to control and results were either too subtle for patient satisfaction or too intense and resulted in burns. With the aim of more precisely controlling the depth to which heat was applied, laser resurfacing technologies, including carbon dioxide and erbium YAG lasers were developed for facial rejuvenation.[13,24–26] In a photothermolytic process, photons from these lasers interacted with dermal water resulting in ablative coagulative disruption of dermal collagen triple helices. An immediate skin tightening ensued, followed by a secondary tightening effect over the next 6 months owing to neocollagenesis and production of elastin and ground substances.[13] Although these technologies provided significant rhytid reduction and superficial skin tightening, they regularly led to an unacceptable degree of postprocedure erythema, swelling, and downtime.[8]

In an attempt to reproduce the results of ablative lasers while reducing downtime and complications, nonablative laser and light technologies were developed. These devices work by photons interacting with a dermal chromophore, such as melanin or hemoglobin.[13] The downtime and recovery from these nonablative technologies was far more tolerable than full ablative lasers, but multiple treatments were often required and the long-term results often fell short of patient expectation.[13,27–29] Additionally, because these technologies rely on interaction with dermal chromophores, they were often unpredictable when used on patients with higher Fitzpatrick skin types and had the potential for long-term complications such as demarcation, pigmentation irregularities, and scarring.[30,31] This limitation sparked the development of skin tightening technologies that were nonablative, did not rely on chromophore interaction, and produced significant skin tightening while minimizing downtime and postoperative edema.

Each type of collagen has an optimal temperature at which remodeling is induced while avoiding destruction.[4] RF energy interaction with collagen has been studied in cornea, joint cartilage, and vascular tissue, and the threshold for collagen denaturation depends on the tissue wherein it resides. This ranges from approximately 60°C to 80°C.[19] RF-based devices produce heating through the application of an electromagnetic current instead of interaction with a chromophore. As electrons shift polarity and move within the targeted tissue, heating is produced through tissue resistance according to Ohms law.[13] The depth of heating depends on several factors, including the tissue's impedance and the frequency of the current.[19]

Early RF devices emitted energy at the skin surface using electrode arrays, which required energy to pass through the epidermis to heat the underlying dermis. This represented an inherent safety limitation, because the threshold temperature for an epidermal burn is roughly 48°C, which is significantly lower than the optimal temperature for dermal collagen contraction, roughly 60°C to 65°C.[19] As a result, aggressive skin cooling and multiple short duration treatments were required. Surface temperature thresholds also limited the depth to which electrothermal energy could penetrate into the dermis, because increasing the RF power (and thereby depth) would necessarily increase the heat delivered to the skin surface.

To circumvent these issues, transcutaneous (or microneedle) RF technologies were developed that delivered energy directly into the dermis, bypassing the epidermal–dermal junction. In this technique, a fractionated tip or array of needles is inserted in the skin, each with parallel rows of bipolar electrodes, creating closed circuits among the pins. The density of the pins and amount of energy controls the intensity of ablation. The pattern of dermal injury is minimal at the epidermis, and increases in size as the RF energy descends to deeper layers of the dermis. This technique results in a lower potential for skin surface injury while allowing for higher temperatures to be delivered to dermal collagen. Additionally, because these RF technologies do not depend on interaction with chromophores to create heat, they deliver a more even and widespread energy distribution that is safe on all skin types without risk for hyperpigmentation.[32,33]

Microneedle RF technologies safely and successfully produce modest skin tightening and rhytid reduction by heating the papillary and reticular dermis.[13,34–37] RF energy has also been shown to decrease elastotic material in the upper dermis and induce reorientation of elastic fibers within the papillary and upper reticular dermis.[38] Nevertheless, treating conditions resulting from skin laxity, jowling, and platysmal banding requires heating of deeper subdermis that cannot be achieved by RF microneedle technologies alone.[22,39] The dermis and underlying hypodermis create a complex collagen network involving the papillary and reticular dermal layers, fatty, fibrous septi, and underlying fascial layers, all of which act in concert with the more superficial dermal skin layers to create the skin's tone, quality, and durability. Unfortunately, transcutaneous microneedle RF technologies are unable to deliver consistent and measurable heat to the deeper hypodermal layers and their effect is limited to dermal collagenous tissue.[2] Furthermore, subcutaneous, preplatysmal adiposity cannot be addressed with microneedle technologies, which limits their effectiveness in many patients presenting for rejuvenation.

DEVELOPMENT OF SUBDERMAL ENERGY DELIVERY DEVICES

Recently, subdermal energy delivery technologies have been introduced which simultaneously ablate subcutaneous fat, as well as tighten the overlying skin.

Subdermal Laser-Assisted Lipolysis

Since the first multicenter study of LAL,[40] the technique has been updated and advanced by multiple groups of investigators, including the development of devices that introduce laser energy directly into subdermal tissue using fiberoptic lasers.[13,16,41–43] Histologic analysis after these techniques showed coagulation of small blood vessels, rupture of adipocytes, reorganization of the reticular dermis, and coagulation of collagen in fat tissue. A growing base of evidence has since shown that subdermal LAL can induce moderate tissue skin contraction without ablation of the epidermal–dermal junction, as well as a decrease in subcutaneous fat volume.[44]

The physics, quantification, and safety of subdermal thermal energy delivery was later defined by DiBernardo and colleagues[45] in an investigation of subdermal LAL using fiberoptic 1064 nm, 1320 nm, and multiplex lasers (Smart Lipo, Cynosure Inc., Westford, MA). DiBernardo and associates showed that administering laser energy directly into the subdermal space (5 mm below the skin surface) and heating the subdermis to 50°C to 55°C resulted in a nonablative, coagulative disruption of the deep reticular collagen fibers.[45] DiBernardo and coworkers also found that heating the subdermis to 50°C to 55°C correlated with epidermal temperatures between 40°C to 42°C, and that epidermal and dermal injuries typically occurred when surface temperatures increased beyond 47°C.

Subsequently, the same authors released a preliminary report on skin shrinkage and increased elasticity as a result of multiwavelength LAL,[46] followed by a randomized, blinded, split abdomen study showing that LAL induced greater mean skin shrinkage and tightening versus SAL alone at one and 3 months after treatment.[47] Furthermore, LAL allowed for a small diameter cannula, which permitted treatment to superficial areas such as the face and neck where it is difficult to remove fat and where irregularities are common after treatment.

Nevertheless, relatively slow treatment speeds, poor control of uniform heating, and a risk profile of burns limited the usefulness of LAL, and inspired further development of alternative energy-based lipolysis devices.

Radiofrequency-Assisted Liposuction/Lipolysis

In 2009, Paul and Mulholland[3] introduced RF-assisted liposuction/lipolysis (RFAL), a novel method for body contouring using a bipolar subdermal (percutaneous) RF device (BodyTite system, Invasix Ltd, Yokneam, Israel). The BodyTite system consists of a bipolar handpiece that includes a subcutaneous RF delivery probe to treat the septofascial and fasciocutaneous structures of the subdermis, and an external electrode that glides along the skin surface, functioning as the bipolar return electrode and as a transepidermal nonfractionated RF energy delivery system for the papillary and reticular dermis.[3] The investigators examined 40 lipoplasty zones in 20 patients, comparing the effectiveness and safety profile of RFAL to LAL (Smart Lipo, Cynosure Inc.) and standard power-assisted liposuction. LAL demonstrated relatively poor surface temperature uniformity, wherein epidermal hot spots of up to 47°C were noted during treatment while a significant part of the thermal zone was cold, below 35°C. This condition led to either early cessation of treatment resulting in lack of uniform heating, poor skin contraction, inconsistent results, or created a high risk for burns if additional energy was applied. In contrast, the temperature, impedance, and power controls of the BodyTite device enabled sustained RF delivery at subnecrotic thermal levels that were reached more quickly than with LAL. The result was twice the heating uniformity as LAL and facilitated longer treatment times at critical target temperatures. Other advantages over LAL included strong defragmentation of fat cells and coagulation of blood vessels in the treated zone, decreasing bleeding and bruising, significant tissue contraction, and retraction of the entire subcutaneous fibrous and dermal matrix.[3]

In a follow-up study, Paul and colleagues[4] presented results from a series of patients undergoing RFAL for body contouring and proposed the mechanism for RFAL by comparing the threshold temperature and contraction levels of 3 different types of ex vivo collagenous tissues, namely, adipose tissue with septal and reticular connective tissue, dermis, and fascia. The strongest contraction response was observed in adipose tissue containing septal connective tissue and reticular collagen fibers encasing fat cells. The contraction temperature threshold was the highest for dermis at 81.9°C, while the septa with adipose tissue and dermis contracted at 61.5°C and 69.4°C, respectively. These results reaffirmed that only transcutaneous, subdermal delivery of RF could heat the fascia and septa to necessarily high enough temperatures while avoiding epidermal burns. Patients demonstrated statistically significantly greater tissue tightening than reported with other energy-based liposuction technologies and the overall area contraction was more substantial than linear contraction. Because the dermis was not routinely heated to defined threshold temperatures during treatment, the investigators confirmed that skin tightening and elasticity change after RFAL was not the result of dermal collagen contraction, but instead is the result of subdermal tissue contraction of vertical and oblique fibrous adipose matrices[4] (**Fig. 3**).

The principles of body contouring with RFAL, developed by Paul and Mulholland, were then applied face and neck using a newer, smaller bipolar RF device (FaceTite, Invasix Ltd).[48] Forty-two patients with face and neck skin laxity were treated with the FaceTite hand piece powered by the Body-Tite platform using more conservative temperature thresholds than with body RFAL (38°C–40°C vs 40°C–42°C for body RFAL). The result was clinically significant tightening and lifting of the brow, lower lid, cheek, and neck beginning at 3 to 4 weeks and continuing over 6 months. Punch biopsies

were taken immediately after treatment, revealing localized coagulative necrosis of subcutaneous fat, collagen, and fibrous tissue coagulation at the dermis–fat junction and restructuring of the reticular dermis without disruption the fasciocutaneous blood supply. No complications were reported, including no hyperpigmentation in patients with Fitzpatrick skin types IV or V.

Subdermal monopolar radiofrequency

The preliminary success of the FaceTite system soon invited new competitive technologies into the percutaneous RF landscape. Prior work by Royo de la Torre and colleagues[49] showed that variability in tissue density and conductivity in the subdermis can quickly and unpredictably increase subdermal temperatures during transcutaneous RF, resulting in pain or burns. With these data in mind, Key introduced the concept of thermistor-controlled percutaneous RF using a monopolar subdermal RF system that included novel real-time subdermal and epidermal temperature monitoring systems (ThermiTight, ThermiAesthetics, Southlake, TX).[2] During the preliminary investigation in 18 patients, the investigators reported a weak linear dependence between subdermal and epidermal temperatures, similar to the results of Royo de la Torre and colleagues.[49] As such, the monopolar ThermiTight device was developed to

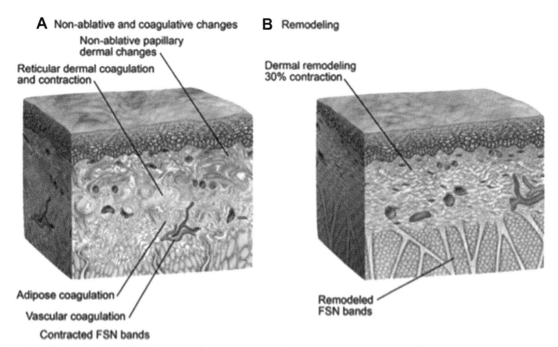

Fig. 3. Effects after FaceTite. (*A*) Immediate changes to the dermis and subdermis following percutaneous radiofrequency treatment. (*B*) Collagen remodeling in months following percutaneous radiofrequency treatment. FSN, Fibroseptal network. (*From* Mulholland RS. Nonexcisional, minimally invasive rejuvenation of the neck. Clin Plast Surg 2014;41(1):23; with permission.)

include a thermistor, which is a temperature sensing element at the distal tip of the treatment probe that detects changes in resistance when exposed to small temperature changes. The thermistor constantly modulates the RF output current during treatment, allowing for precise and consistent subdermal temperatures to be reached for longer durations without the development of hot spots or burns. Mean and median subdermal temperatures were 55.4°C and 55°C, respectively. The ThermiTight system was integrated with a forward looking infrared (FLIR) camera that continuously monitors epidermal temperatures of during treatment and displays them for the physician to view. The FLIR temperature readings were compared with a standard external handheld infrared laser thermometer, which found a significant difference in readings, thus supporting the use of the FLIR camera. FLIR monitors the entire field, not just 1 spot. No complications were reported in any of the patients.

The clinical usefulness of the ThermiTight system was then evaluated in 35 patients undergoing treatment of submental and jowl skin laxity.[2] Subsurface temperature settings were set between 50°C and 60°C and the clinical endpoint for a particular treatment site was defined at an epidermal temperature of 42°C. Two blinded reviewers graded patient photographs at baseline and 30 days postoperatively on a 4-point skin laxity scale. Seventy-four percent of patients demonstrated clinical improvements in skin laxity, with a mean change of −0.78/4.00 ($P <$ .001). Mild erythema was noted in some patients that lasted less than 12 hours and no complications were reported.

DEVICES

As of this writing, only 2 percutaneous RF devices have been cleared by the US Food and Drug Administration for face and neck treatment—the ThermiTight (ThermiAesthetics) and FaceTite (InMode Corporation, Toronto, Canada).

The FaceTite system consists of a solid, silicon-coated, 1.8-mm diameter, 13-cm long, RF-emitting probe with a bullet-shaped plastic tip connected to a console containing the RF card, electronics, and a central processing unit with graphical user interface (**Fig. 4**). In this bipolar system, the RF current flows unidirectionally from the internal/subdermal probe out to the external electrode, which glides along the epidermal surface in tandem with the RF-emitting internal electrode. The external electrode contains a series of sensors that relay information to the console and CPU, including high and low soft tissue impedance sensors and epidermal contact and thermal sensors. The epidermal temperature is monitored and sampled 10 times per millisecond and the RF energy is turned off

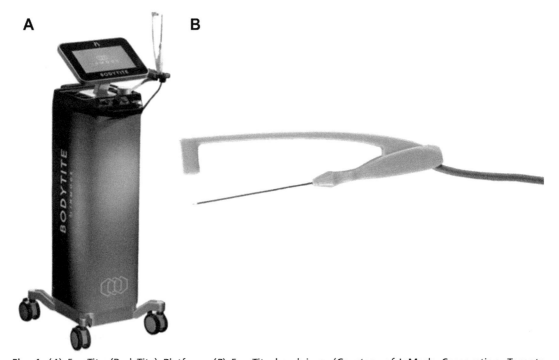

Fig. 4. (A) FaceTite (BodyTite) Platform. (B) FaceTite handpiece. (*Courtesy of* InMode Corporation, Toronto, Canada.)

when the selected therapeutic end point is achieved and turned on when epidermis decreases to 0.1°C below the target epidermal temperature. The platform gives audio feedback in the form of bell signals when the temperature is within 2°C of goal temperature and when goal temperature has been reached.

The ThermiTight system consists of solid, blunt, 18-G monopolar subdermal RF emitting probes that vary in length from 5 to 20 cm long from handpiece to distal tip (**Fig. 5**). The handpiece is connected to the Thermi console, where the subdermal temperature treatment goal is set by the user. This monopolar device produces 3-dimensional volumetric heating as the current flows from the handpiece to the grounding pad, which is placed on the patient. The energy confinement at 50°C is limited to roughly a 3-mm radius from the treatment probe tip. Safety features include the treatment probe thermistor (described in detail elsewhere in this article), as well as constant epidermal temperature monitoring via a FLIR camera system.

PROCEDURE DESCRIPTION

The patient is placed in a seated position with the lower face and neck exposed. Informed consent is obtained and pretreatment photos are taken. A wheal of lidocaine, 1%, with epinephrine 1:100,000 is raised bilaterally underneath each earlobe and in the central submental crease. A 16-G needle is then used to create 3 pilot hole openings in the skin at the site of prior lidocaine injection, piercing through the dermis and entering the subcutaneous tissue. The lower face and neck are then sterilely prepped and draped. Tumescent anesthesia (10 mL lidocaine, 1%; 1.5 mL sodium bicarbonate, 8.4%; and 0.4 mL epinephrine 1:1000 in 100 mL 0.9% normal saline) is then introduced through the 3 previously made needle openings using a tumescent fluid infusion cannula. Typically, 80 to 100 mL of tumescent is used to treat the entire lower face and neck with approximately 20 mL injected per neck treatment area (eg, left neck, left jowl, right neck, right jowl, and central neck/submentum). Tumescent fluid is

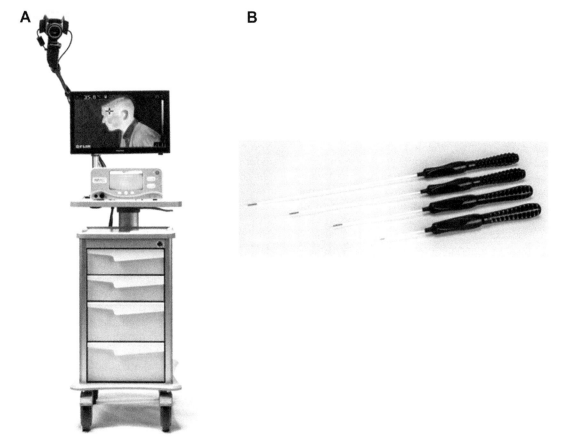

Fig. 5. (A) ThermiTight Platform. (B) ThermiTight handpieces. (*Courtesy of* InMode Corporation, Toronto, Canada.)

a critical component to the procedure. The water in the tumescent fluid aids in good RF conductivity, provides adequate clearance within the subcutaneous fat space required for the instrument to travel, and provides a secondary source of heat transfer heat after the application of the RF energy has been completed. Additionally, when using the FaceTite system, the turgor of the overlying soft tissues provided by the tumescent fluid ensure satisfactory coupling of the external probe to the skin.[50]

In general, both the ThermiTight and FaceTite procedures have been proven safe and well-tolerated in office settings under local anesthesia. Some patients and physicians prefer the use of selective nerve blocks or general anesthesia, particularly if additional surgical or minimally invasive procedures are to be combined with percutaneous RF treatments. Oral analgesia in the form of benzodiazepines are also commonly used. Once adequate anesthesia is obtained, the RF probe is inserted into the left infraauricular pilot hole and advanced/retracted subcutaneously at alternating angles to create subcutaneous tunnels through which the probe will travel when the RF energy is initiated. The RF probe is then inserted along the inferior mandibular border completely to its hub and the device energy is activated. The probe is withdrawn 1 cm at a time, delivering energy for approximately 5 seconds in each spot before being withdrawn each additional centimeter. Next, the probe is fanned across the left neck by inserting the probe and then applying the energy as the probe is continuously withdrawn. Once the left neck is completed, the left jowl area is next treated. It is important to apply the probe immediately subcutaneous in this area and not dive deeper into the jowl fat because the terminal branches of the marginal mandibular branch of the facial nerve are in close proximity. Some users have advocated for mapping of the marginal mandibular nerve preoperatively with a transcutaneous nerve stimulator; however, this step has not been necessary in these authors' experience. Once the left jowl area is completed, the right neck, right jowl, and central/submental areas are then treated in sequence.

Treatment time is approximately 7 to 10 minutes per lateral neck area, 1 to 2 minutes per jowl area, and 3 to 5 minutes in the central neck zone. In general, a treatment zone surface area of 3 cm^2 is treated every 2 minutes, with total treatment times between 25 and 38 minutes yielding optimal results.[51] It is important to understand, however, that subdermal and epidermal surface temperatures, not time, define the treatment durations within each area. Usually, epidermal temperature

limit is set between 38°C and 42°C, whereas the subdermal temperature goal is set between 50°C and 65°C depending on the user and the treatment area.

The techniques for ThermiTight (Video 1) and FaceTite (Video 2) are essentially the same, with the addition of ultrasound gel being applied to the skin when using the FaceTite device to decrease friction from the external receiving electrode (see Video 2). Once the procedure is completed, a microliposuction cannula is used to aspirate any liquefied fat from the treatment areas because this can increase postprocedure irritation and/or inflammation if left in situ. This measure is generally recommended if more than 20 mL of liquefied fat is expected to be aspirated. A single 6-0 fast-absorbing gut suture is used to close the port holes if liposuction was performed; otherwise, they are allowed to heal by secondary intention. The patient is discharged with a neck compression garment to be worn for 24 to 48 hours, then nightly for 1 week. In the authors' experience, postprocedural opiate pain medications have not been required and pain is well-controlled with over-the-counter analgesics.

DISCUSSION

As of 2011, a person is turning 60 year old every 10 seconds. In 2011, one-fourth of the US population is between 42 and 60 years old, representing nearly 100 million people with skin laxity who may benefit aesthetically from an excisional surgical procedure.[52] Nevertheless, fewer than 180,000 excisional surgeries on the face and neck were performed in the United States in 2017, indicating that only 1% to 2% of patients with cervical skin laxity actually present for an excisional procedure.[8] Since the early 2000s, there has been an explosion of new minimally invasive and noninvasive skin tightening technologies in the United States and internationally. Many aging patients today are willing to accept less significant results with fewer complications and shorter recovery versus more effective invasive surgical procedures. Additionally, the age at which patients present for rejuvenation continues to decrease, with 49% of cosmetic procedures in the United States being performed on patients 20 to 54 years old.[6] The average millennial will take 25,000 selfies in their lifetime and are more aware of their appearance to the world than any preceding generation.[50] In these increasingly younger and more savvy populations, surgical neck rejuvenation has been stagnant or decreasing in recent years, with 2000 fewer neck lifts performed in 2017 than 2016 (a 4% decrease). In the same time frame, minimally invasive fat reduction and skin tightening, including in the neck, has increased by 7% and 9%, respectively, with nearly 700,000 combined procedures performed in 2017. It is, therefore, of critical importance for plastic surgeons to keep abreast of and master the wide variety of alternatives to excisional procedures to treat the lower face and neck.

Percutaneous RF technologies deliver significantly higher power with greater energy transfer efficiency than LAL or other energy systems. In percutaneous RF systems, optimal temperatures are delivered to the whole volume of treated tissue, not only the superficial subdermal layer, and can heat deep adipose and subcutaneous tissue to much higher temperatures without compromising skin safety.[4] Histologic analysis immediately after treatment with percutaneous RF reveals coagulative necrosis of the subdermal fat layer and the deep reticular dermis, as well as nonablative coagulation of the papillary dermis. Coagulation of small blood vessels in the hypodermis is also evident, which may decrease postoperative ecchymosis.[50] Skin biopsies at 12 months after the procedure show normal dermal architecture with healthy collagen and elastin fibers in the deep reticular dermis and no evidence of scar tissue or abnormal collagen fibers.[4]

Published results from percutaneous RF treatments have generally shown up to a 25% area contraction at 6 months and 35% to 60% achieved at 1 year, statistically significantly higher than results reported with other energy emitting liposuction or skin tightening technologies.[4,8,13,46,50,53] This level of skin contraction is often considered a successful aesthetic outcome in patients who might otherwise have required an excisional procedure. The success of these procedures also increases the potential patient population who may not have skin laxity severe enough to warrant a standard excisional operation, but will likely have a poor aesthetic outcome with liposuction alone owing to deficient elasticity of the overlying skin.[50] The authors refer to these patients as "tweeners"—patients whose cervical rejuvenation mandates a treatment that falls in between that an excisional procedure and of noninvasive skin resurfacing with or without liposuction. Results at 6 months for a typical patient treated with FaceTite are shown (**Fig. 6**).

The national mean physicians fee for a surgical face/neck lift is $7448, whereas the average fee for noninvasive fat reduction is $1481 and $2060 for nonsurgical skin tightening. In contrast, the average physicians fee for one ThermiTight or FaceTite treatment between is $3000 and $4500.[54] Although the majority of percutaneous RF treatments are one-time only procedures, providing these treatments can enhance a surgeon's downstream operative volume, because some of these patients will ultimately require excisional procedures and a trusting relationship has already been established between the surgeon and patient. This finding is supported by recent data indicating approximately 45% of patients who underwent cosmetic procedures in 2017 had undergone prior cosmetic procedures, either surgical, noninvasive, or minimally invasive.[6] The senior author often discounts an excisional procedure for patients who have previously undergone percutaneous RF treatment in his practice. The results of percutaneous RF treatments can also be enhanced by providing additional nonsurgical procedures, such as RF microneedling, neuromodulators, dermal fillers, or laser/chemical skin resurfacing. Some surgeons have also advocated using percutaneous RF devices to undermine skin flaps of the neck and lower face as part of rhytidectomy,[3,8] whereas others may offer these treatments to patients after rhytidectomy to maintain skin tightening results. Early publications with ThermiTight studied the effect on facial nerve ablation for treatment glabellar frown lines and platysmal banding, although the practical applications never developed for these indications.

African Americans and Hispanics underwent 1.6 million and 1.9 million cosmetic procedures in 2017, respectively, a 17% and 16% increase, respectively, from the year prior. This increase is in contrast with an 8% increase among Caucasians, who underwent 12.3 million procedures. Because percutaneous RF treatments are chromophore independent, they are safe and effective in patients with darker skin tones, and this characteristic represents an opportunity to provide energy-based skin tightening for these populations who are increasingly seeking cosmetic cervicofacial rejuvenation.

Most patients seeking treatment for cervical rejuvenation are between 45 and 55 years old, roughly 60% of whom are considered by treating physicians to be suitable candidates for treatment with percutaneous RF technology.[51] In recent expert consensus panel and physician surveys on percutaneous temperature-controlled RF treatments, nearly 90% agreed that procedures with these devices in appropriate patients can safely and effectively achieve skin tightening and fat reduction of the submental tissue and jowls. In these patients, 95% of physicians agreed that percutaneous RF treatments deliver comprehensive skin tightening and 85% agreed skin tightening continues to be evident 6 months after a single treatment.[51]

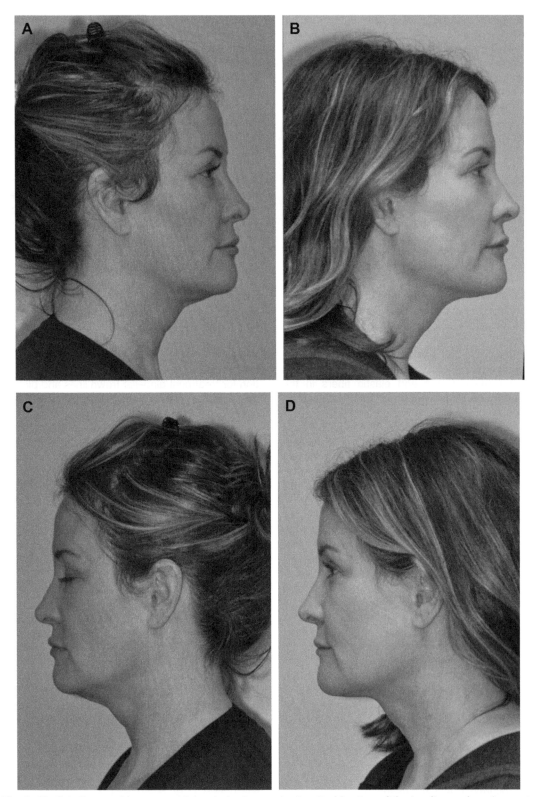

Fig. 6. (*A, C*) A 48-year-old woman with cervical submental adiposity, blunting of the jaw line and cervicomental angle, mild jowling, and mild skin ptosis. (*B, D*) Six months after FaceTite procedure to the lower face and neck.

Although standardized treatment parameters, temperature protocols, contraindications, and preoperative and postoperative analgesic regimens are still being developed, a best practices treatment algorithm has been published for subdermal monopolar radiofrequency with ThermiTight (**Box 1**).

Patient selection is critical to achieving optimal outcomes with percutaneous RF treatments. Unsuitable candidates include women during pregnancy; patients with collagen vascular diseases, autoimmune diseases, or acute infections; patients with cochlear and neurostimulator implants; and patients with morbid conditions that could make them unsuitable for the procedure. For patients with an external pacemaker, implantable defibrillator, or monitoring equipment, an attending cardiologist should be consulted before undertaking the procedure. All implanted devices should be evaluated for contraindications from the manufacturer. In addition, patients with preplatysmal adiposity and skin laxity must be distinguished

---

Box 1
Best practices guidelines for scalable multifunction RF with ThermiTight

- Candidates for scalable multifunction RF
  - Mild to moderate skin laxity.
  - Fat reduction of the submentum, lateral neck, mandibular border, and jowl lateral to the nasolabial fold.
- Preparation
  - Clean the area of insertion with 4% chlorhexidine solution or betadine.
  - Administer diluted lidocaine solution via the subdermal cannula using a double Klein Solution (ie, 0.2% concentration).
  - Optional: Map the marginal mandibular nerve using a peripheral nerve stimulator.
- Procedure
  - Divide the neck into 3 zones, namely, the paramedian, right, and left lateral zones.
  - Insert the electrode fully.
  - Avoid skin contact with the hub.
  - Wait for the actual temperature to reach the set temperature. Subsurface temperature target is set between 55°C and 56°C and epidermal temperature is not to exceed 46°C.
  - Monitor the epidermal temperature with the external infrared FLIR camera throughout the procedure.
  - Slowly withdraw the electrode approximately 0.5 to 1.0 cm per second.
  - Keep the actual temperature within 3°C to 5°C of the set temperature.
  - Repeat liner strokes in a fanning manner until the area has been treated, reaching the clinical end points with each stroke.
- Clinical end point
  - The skin temperature should reach between 42°C and 46°C over the entire area treated.
  - The entire area must be a uniform color (yellow-white color on the infrared monitor); use the FLIR default color scheme.
  - The actual temperature and set temperature should remain within 3° of each other throughout the entire procedure.
- Preventing complications
  - Avoid tenting the skin.
  - Avoid catching the dermis with the cannula.
  - Avoid end-hitting distal skin with the tip of the cannula.
  - Monitor the skin temperature and cool with saline-soaked swabs for skin heated to more than 46°C.

Data from Kinney BM, Andriessen A, DiBernardo BE, et al. Use of a controlled subdermal radio frequency thermistor for treating the aging neck: Consensus recommendations. J Cosmet Laser Ther 2017;19(8):444–50.

from those significant subplatysmal fat, which also compromises the appearance of a youthful neck, but is more difficult to treat without an excisional procedure, and will not respond as ideally to percutaneous RF treatments. Reported thermal injuries are in the 1% range, with most occurring within the first 10 to 15 cases.[3,50] Nevertheless, when a percutaneous RF treatment does result in a burn, it is by definition full thickness, and often will require surgical excision and management.

SUMMARY

Percutaneous RF technologies have recently been introduced to safely and effectively ablate subcutaneous fat and tighten skin by delivering energy directly into the subdermal space, targeting the upper dermal collagen network, the deeper fascial layer, and fibrofatty septum. Ideal candidates for percutaneous RF treatments have early jowling or jaw line blunting, mild to moderate marionette lines, early neck tissue laxity, or minimal to moderate submental adiposity. These patients are considered by the authors as tweeners, whose cervical rejuvenation mandates a treatment that falls in between that of an excisional procedure and of noninvasive skin resurfacing with or without liposuction. In these patients, a 30% to 40% area contraction at 6 months and 40% to 50% at 1 year is common after treatment and is statistically significantly higher than results reported with other energy emitting liposuction or skin tightening technologies. Percutaneous RF treatments are marketed to patients as a one-time no sutures, no scalpels, no surgery procedure performed in the office under local anesthesia with long-lasting effects and minimal downtime. Percutaneous RF treatments can drive practice volume by recruiting patients who may not have otherwise presented for cervical rejuvenation owing to fear of surgery and because some patients treated with these technologies will ultimately present for excisional procedures later in life. Additionally, percutaneous RF treatments can be combined with additional skin resurfacing procedures such as RF microneedling or CO_2 laser, or with neuromodulators and/or dermal fillers. Percutaneous RF is also chromophore independent, which allows for safe and effective treatment of patients with darker skin types, who are increasingly seeking cosmetic cervicofacial rejuvenation.

SUPPLEMENTARY DATA

Supplementary data related to this article can be found online at https://doi.org/10.1016/j.fsc.2019.03.003.

REFERENCES

1. Key DJ. Comprehensive thermoregulation for the purpose of skin tightening using a novel radiofrequency treatment device: a preliminary report. J Drugs Dermatol 2014;13(2):185–9.
2. Key DJ. Integration of thermal imaging with subsurface radiofrequency thermistor heating for the purpose of skin tightening and contour improvement: a retrospective review of clinical efficacy. J Drugs Dermatol 2014;13(12):1485–9.
3. Paul M, Mulholland RS. A new approach for adipose tissue treatment and body contouring using radiofrequency-assisted liposuction. Aesthetic Plast Surg 2009;33(5):687–94.
4. Paul M, Blugerman G, Kreindel M, et al. Three-dimensional radiofrequency tissue tightening: a proposed mechanism and applications for body contouring. Aesthetic Plast Surg 2011;35(1):87–95.
5. Locketz GD, Bloom JD. Percutaneous radiofrequency lower face and neck tightening technique. JAMA Facial Plast Surg 2018. https://doi.org/10.1001/jamafacial.2018.0917.
6. American Society of Plastic Surgeons. 2017 Plastic Surgery Statistics Report. 2017.
7. American Society of Dermatologic Surgery. 2018 ASDS consumer survey on cosmetic dermatologic procedures. 2018.
8. Mulholland RS. Nonexcisional, minimally invasive rejuvenation of the neck. Clin Plast Surg 2014;41(1):11–31.
9. Kim YH, Cha SM, Naidu S, et al. Analysis of postoperative complications for superficial liposuction: a review of 2398 cases. Plast Reconstr Surg 2011;127(2):863–71.
10. Illouz Y-G. Surgical remodeling of the silhouette by aspiration lipolysis or selective lipectomy. Aesthetic Plast Surg 1985;9(1):7–21.
11. Klein JA. Anesthesia for liposuction in dermatologic surgery. J Dermatol Surg Oncol 1988;14(10):1124–32.
12. Gasparotti M. Superficial liposuction: a new application of the technique for aged and flaccid skin. Aesthetic Plast Surg 1992;16(2):141–53.
13. Mulholland RS. Radio frequency energy for noninvasive and minimally invasive skin tightening. Clin Plast Surg 2011;38(3):437–48.
14. Parlette EC, Kaminer ME. Laser-assisted liposuction: here's the skinny. Semin Cutan Med Surg 2008;27(4):259–63.
15. Heymans O, Castus P, Grandjean FX, et al. Liposuction: review of the techniques, innovations and applications. Acta Chir Belg 2006;106(6):647–53.
16. Goldman A, Gotkin RH. Laser-assisted liposuction. Clin Plast Surg 2009;36(2):241–53.
17. Mann MW, Palm MD, Sengelmann RD. New advances in liposuction technology. Semin Cutan Med Surg 2008;27(1):72–82.

18. Fredricks S. Analysis and introduction of a technology: ultrasound-assisted lipoplasty task force. Clin Plast Surg 1999;26(2):187–204, vii.
19. Pritzker RN, Robinson DM. Updates in noninvasive and minimally invasive skin tightening. Semin Cutan Med Surg 2014;33(4):182–7.
20. Sieber DA, Kenkel JM. Noninvasive methods for lower facial rejuvenation. Clin Plast Surg 2018; 45(4):571–84.
21. Arnoczky SP, Aksan A. Thermal modification of connective tissues: basic science considerations and clinical implications. J Am Acad Orthop Surg 2000; 8(5):305–13.
22. Gold MH. Update on tissue tightening. J Clin Aesthet Dermatol 2010;3(5):36–41.
23. Locketz GD, Bloom BD. Combining radiofrequency systems to treat the neck. Int J Aesthetic Anti-Aging Med 2018;6(2).
24. Fitzpatrick RE, Goldman MP, Satur NM, et al. Pulsed carbon dioxide laser resurfacing of photoaged facial skin. Arch Dermatol 1996;132(4): 395–402.
25. Fitzpatrick RE. CO2 laser resurfacing. Dermatol Clin 2001;19(3):443–51, viii.
26. Sapijaszko MJA, Zachary CB. Er:YAG laser skin resurfacing. Dermatol Clin 2002;20(1):87–96.
27. Goldberg DJ. Nonablative dermal remodeling: does it really work? Arch Dermatol 2002;138(10): 1366–8.
28. Sadick NS. Update on non-ablative light therapy for rejuvenation: a review. Lasers Surg Med 2003;32(2): 120–8.
29. Hardaway CA, Ross EV. Nonablative laser skin remodeling. Dermatol Clin 2002;20(1):97–111, ix.
30. Brunner E, Adamson PA, Harlock JN, et al. Laser facial resurfacing: patient survey of recovery and results. J Otolaryngol 2000;29(6):377–81.
31. Nanni CA, Alster TS. Complications of carbon dioxide laser resurfacing. An evaluation of 500 patients. Dermatol Surg 1998;24(3):315–20.
32. Man J, Goldberg DJ. Safety and efficacy of fractional bipolar radiofrequency treatment in Fitzpatrick skin types V–VI. J Cosmet Laser Ther 2012;87(6): 179–83.
33. Lee HS, Lee DH, Won CH, et al. Fractional rejuvenation using a novel bipolar radiofrequency system in Asian skin. Dermatol Surg 2011;37(11):1611–9.
34. Sukal SA, Geronemus RG. Thermage: the nonablative radiofrequency for rejuvenation. Clin Dermatol 2008;26(6):602–7.
35. Bitter P, Stephen Mulholland R. Report of a new technique for enhanced non-invasive skin rejuvenation using a dual mode pulsed light and radiofrequency energy source: selective radio-thermolysis. J Cosmet Dermatol 2002;1(3):142–3.
36. Fitzpatrick R, Geronemus R, Goldberg D, et al. Multicenter study of noninvasive radiofrequency for periorbital tissue tightening. Lasers Surg Med 2003;33(4):232–42.
37. Dover JS, Zelickson B, 14-Physician Multispecialty Consensus Panel. Results of a survey of 5,700 patient monopolar radiofrequency facial skin tightening treatments: assessment of a low-energy multiple-pass technique leading to a clinical end point algorithm. Dermatol Surg 2007;33(8):900–7.
38. El-Domyati M, El-Ammawi TS, Medhat W, et al. Radiofrequency facial rejuvenation: evidence-based effect. J Am Acad Dermatol 2011;64(3):524–35.
39. Woolery-Lloyd H, Kammer JN. Skin tightening. Curr Probl Dermatol 2011;42:147–52.
40. Apfelberg DB. Results of multicenter study of laser-assisted liposuction. Clin Plast Surg 1996;23(4): 713–9.
41. Goldman A. Submental Nd:Yag laser-assisted liposuction. Lasers Surg Med 2006;38(3):181–4.
42. Woodhall KE, Saluja R, Khoury J, et al. A comparison of three separate clinical studies evaluating the safety and efficacy of laser-assisted lipolysis using 1,064, 1,320nm, and a combined 1,064/ 1,320nm multiplex device. Lasers Surg Med 2009; 41(10):774–8.
43. Ichikawa K, Miyasaka M, Tanaka R, et al. Histologic evaluation of the pulsed Nd:YAG laser for laser lipolysis. Lasers Surg Med 2005;36(1):43–6.
44. Kim KH, Geronemus RG. Laser lipolysis using a novel 1,064 nm Nd:YAG Laser. Dermatol Surg 2006;32(2):241–8 [discussion: 247].
45. DiBernardo BE, Reyes J, Chen B. Evaluation of tissue thermal effects from 1064/1320-nm laser-assisted lipolysis and its clinical implications. J Cosmet Laser Ther 2009;11(2):62–9.
46. DiBernardo B. Journal JR-A surgery, 2009 undefined. Preliminary report: evaluation of skin tightening after laser-assisted liposuction. Available at: academic.oup.com. Accessed November 4, 2018.
47. DiBernardo BE. Randomized, blinded split abdomen study evaluating skin shrinkage and skin tightening in laser-assisted liposuction versus liposuction control. Aesthet Surg J 2010;30(4):593–602.
48. Ahn DH, Mulholland RS, Duncan D, et al. Non-excisional face and neck tightening using a novel subdermal radiofrequency thermo-coagulative device. J Cosmet Dermatological Sci Appl 2011;1:141–6.
49. Royo de la Torre J, Moreno-Moraga J, Muñoz E, et al. Multisource, phase-controlled radiofrequency for treatment of skin laxity: correlation between clinical and in-vivo confocal microscopy results and real-time thermal changes. J Clin Aesthet Dermatol 2011;4(1):28–35.
50. Theodorou SJ, Del Vecchio D, Chia CT. Soft tissue contraction in body contouring with radiofrequency-assisted liposuction: a treatment gap solution. Aesthet Surg J 2018;38(suppl_2): S74–83.

51. Kinney BM, Andriessen A, DiBernardo BE, et al. Use of a controlled subdermal radio frequency thermistor for treating the aging neck: consensus recommendations. J Cosmet Laser Ther 2017; 19(8):444–50.

52. U.S. Census Bureau. QuickFacts: United States. Available at: https://www.census.gov/quickfacts/fact/ table/US/PST045217#PST045217. Accessed October 31, 2018.

53. Duncan DI. Nonexcisional tissue tightening. Aesthet Surg J 2013;33(8):1154–66.

54. Reviews of Cosmetic Treatments, Surgery, Doctors - RealSelf. Available at: https://www.realself.com/. Accessed November 1, 2018.

Microfat and Nanofat
When and Where These Treatments Work

Jordan Rihani, MD

KEYWORDS

- Nanofat • Microfat • Facial volumization • Facial rejuvenation
- Adipose-derived mesenchymal stem cells • Fat grafting • Injectable filler

KEY POINTS

- Newer fat-grafting techniques have decreased many of the original drawbacks of fat-grafting procedures.
- Adipose tissue contains large stores of mesenchymal stem cells that are showing great promise in bioregenerative medicine.
- Injection of nanofat combined with microfat seems to offer improvement in skin texture as well as structural volumization.
- Basic principles of microfat and nanofat are reviewed, as well as a description of injection technique.

INTRODUCTION

Although fat and dermal-fat grafting has been performed for over 50 years[1] and the injection of fat grafts have been performed nearly 30 years,[2] the popularity of facial fat grafting has remained relatively stable. On the contrary, since U.S. Food and Drug Administration approval, the hyaluronic acid filler market has seen an explosive, upward climb.[3] Behind this trend is an increasing awareness by both patients and providers about the important role of volume loss in facial aging. Bone, fat, and muscle loss share equal roles with loss of skin elasticity in the aging process.[4]

The injectable filler market today is a 3 billion dollar industry and includes a variety of products including hyaluronic acid (HA), poly-L-lactic acid, calcium hydroxylapatite, and polymethyl methacrylate. With the ease of use of these products, lack of donor site morbidity, predictable outcome, and the reversibility of HA fillers, it is easy to see

why this market has grown so much over the last 13 years. However, many patients are searching for longer-lasting, more natural solutions than the 9 to 12 month results afforded by most fillers currently available on the market. For these reasons, many have returned to using fat grafting as a solution for many of those shortcomings.

The theoretic draw to fat transfer is easy to see—it seems more "natural" to patients as an autologous graft, it is not price restricted at high volumes, and it is capable of producing long-term results. However, we also must consider the potential downsides, which include: donor site morbidity, unpredictability of graft survival,[5,6] graft hypertrophy,[7,8] and exposure to local or general anesthesia for the procedure.[9] When weighted into the discussion, patients tend to sway less often in the direction of fat transfer. However, recent evolution in fat transfer may have sidestepped many of the shortcomings of the original procedure. Discovery of adipose-derived mesenchymal stem cells

Disclosure Statement: The author has nothing to disclose.
Facial Plastic Surgery Institute, 521 West Southlake Boulevard, Suite 175, Southlake, TX 76092, USA
E-mail address: Jordan@rihanimd.com

Facial Plast Surg Clin N Am 27 (2019) 321–330
https://doi.org/10.1016/j.fsc.2019.03.004

(AD-MSCs) and the elucidation of fat survival patterns following grafting have provided insights for improved outcomes. As a result, the original dermal-fat grafts and microlipoinjection techniques[2,10] have been advanced by current techniques of microfat and nanofat,[11,12] which are showing promising results.

It is known that fat undergoes changes in mass throughout the course of our lives. As fat undergoes these changes, the surrounding blood supply and extracellular matrix must be accommodated—a process mediated, not by the adipocytes themselves, but by signaling of the surrounding stromal vascular fraction (SVF) and its interaction with adipocytes. This nucleated cell fraction includes smooth muscle cells, endothelial cells, blood cells, stem cells, and extracellular matrix. The discovery of large quantities of mesenchymal stem cells present in adipose tissue is likely responsible for most of the signaling in these instances.[13] Signaling of vascular endothelial growth factor, for example, in the creation of new endothelial cells and blood vessels is one example. Several studies have shown that these adult stem cells contain multipotent lineages capable of forming other tissues including bone and muscle.[14–16]

Our understanding of adult mesenchymal stem cells and their multipotent capabilities has combined with ease of methods of enzymatic and mechanical harvest from adipose tissue. The excitement has seen an increase in applications of bioregenerative medicine, especially in facial rejuvenation. Most of these precursor cells are found mixed within the adipocyte population in a typical fat harvest. Isolation of these cells occurs in two ways—either enzymatically or mechanically. Although enzymatic isolation of these cells is most efficient in terms of the concentration of cells harvested, the additional time and requirements of this procedure are not always practical in a surgical setting. The second method for obtaining these is through mechanical isolation. Through techniques of fracturing cell bonds and filtration, the SVF can be isolated from harvested fat in acceptable concentrations.[17]

The mechanical isolation of these adult mesenchymal stem cells, popularized by Tonnard,[11] seems to complement our current methods of structural fat grafting with microfat in a way that addresses many of the needs of volume replacement without many of the drawbacks of the original fat-grafting techniques. Furthermore, combining surgical skin excision with volume replacement has created a "sweet spot" for surgeons creating a look that is natural and not overly pulled, on one end of the spectrum, or overly filled, on the other.

WHAT IS MICROFAT AND NANOFAT?

Fat harvested from the body has a multitude of cells. Adipocytes comprise approximately 30% to 70% of the total cells of harvested fat. Other cells include extracellular matrix, endothelial cells, mural cells, fibroblasts, adipose-derived stem cells, and blood cells.[18] These cells provide the surrounding stroma that support and assist growth of adipose tissue and new blood vessel formation. These AD-MSCs are integral during the grafting process and many believe play a more important role in the fat-grafting process than the adipocytes themselves—demonstrated by the debate between host replacement versus cell survival theories.[19]

The debate regarding whether the host replaces all grafted fat cells (host replacement theory) or whether cells survive the grafting process and remain alive to provide the effect of fat grafting (cell survival theory), seems to show evidence for both mechanisms.[20] Arguments include lack of correlation between surviving adipocytes and final grafted volume and presence of necrosis and fibrosis in histologic sections following fat grafting.

Taking these concepts into consideration, the development of methods of isolating the adult mesenchymal stem cells, or SVF, without living adipocytes has been achieved enzymatically and mechanically. Although the focus of this article is on the mechanical isolation of SVF, the reader should also be familiar with the concept of enzymatic isolation. Enzymatic processing uses the addition of proteolytic enzymes that enable in vitro separation of fat cells from the SVF. Enzymatic digestion allows for the isolation of the SVF pellet of AD-MSCs that can be injected in highly concentrated form.

When the process is performed mechanically, adipocytes are fractured through mechanical emulsification and filtration, leaving the viable SVF intact.[17] Although a misnomer, because there are no viable fat cells, the byproduct of this process is known as "nanofat." This method, described by Tonnard, includes mechanical disruption through small-bore luer lock connectors, followed by filtration through a 500-μm filter.[21] This relatively quick process allows isolation of the SVF as well as some nonviable adipocyte cell components.[22,23] The active component, the SVF, promotes endothelial proliferation, collagen creation, and new cell differentiation and creation.

Conversely, microfat, compared with nanofat, does contain whole and viable adipocytes with their surrounding cell milieu. When injected, these adipocytes act like traditional fat grafts—incorporating into the sites of injection. The term "microfat" refers to the small 1-mm holes in the sides of the liposuction cannula, which allows for smaller grafts than the traditional larger fat-harvesting cannulas, usually 2 to 3 mm in size.

Injection of microfat and nanofat is done in conjunction with one another in my practice. Microfat provides the structural support and volumization, whereas nanofat delivers improvement in fine facial rhytids and neocollagenesis in more cosmetically sensitive areas. Preoperative planning and assessment allow volumes that will be set aside for microfat injections and nanofat injections. After setting aside the appropriate volumes of the harvested microfat to be injected, the remainder undergoes a mechanical isolation process to become nanofat. That mechanical isolation method is described in more detail below.

INDICATIONS FOR FAT TRANSFER

Patients needing generalized volume improvement for multiple regions of the face *with adequate supply of donor fat* are candidates for fat transfer. Regions of volume loss are assessed as follows: forehead and glabella, temples, medial and lateral supraorbital region, outer cheek (including the zygoma and preauricular area), infraorbital and medial cheek, nasolabial folds and upper lip, pyriform aperture, anterior chin and prejowl sulcus, and lateral jawline. Patients undergoing facial rejuvenation surgery with adequate donor supply are considered ideal candidates for fat transfer. In some patients with low body mass index, the adequacy of their donor fat volume is a concern and I will typically discuss alternative methods of volumization—such as poly-L-lactic acid.

CONTRAINDICATIONS

Patients who have undergone multiple rounds of previous liposuction to the donor sites from body-contouring procedures may have little usable fat and tend to have a very fibrous composition to harvested fat, making mechanical isolation of nanofat difficult. I also do not typically offer fat transfer to patients under 40 years because of concerns of hypertrophy later in life.

TECHNIQUE
Marking

Preoperative assessment begins in a stepwise fashion through analysis of patient photographs. Volume changes are assessed in the above-mentioned facial regions. Before surgery, areas of volume deficit are carefully marked in the preoperative room with the patient in the sitting position.

This allows assessment before loss of landmarks with the patient lying supine. The chin is carefully marked using the patient's dentition to help delineate the midline to avoid any asymmetry of the chin with volumization and ensure that the maximal volume is achieved at the midline (**Fig. 1**). The iliac crest is also marked and areas of fat harvest are outlined.

Harvest is typically performed from the lateral thigh in female patients, because this tends to be a common location for fat deposition. Additional advantage of the lateral thigh donor site is that it is well tolerated, is safe to harvest, and shows minimal irregularities following harvest. The abdomen and medial thigh can also be used as donor sites, but they are not the first choice, in my opinion. In men, the abdomen tends to be a more reliable source of donor fat.

The patient is positioned supine with arms outward at 45° from the body to allow access to the donor site. Bilateral thigh and hip are prepped from the iliac crest down to the midthigh, which allows access to the fat pad in that region (**Fig. 2**). Tumescent solution is mixed using a 100-mL bag of 0.9% normal saline with 2 mL of 1% plain lidocaine and 0.1 mL of 1:1000 epinephrine. Tumescent is infiltrated using a tumescent infusion cannula affixed to a 60-mL syringe, and the fluid is instilled and equally distributed between both sides. It is recommended that the tumescent solution sit for 15 minutes after injection and before harvest.

Fat harvesting is performed using 60-mL BD syringes with a Tonnard fat harvester cannula

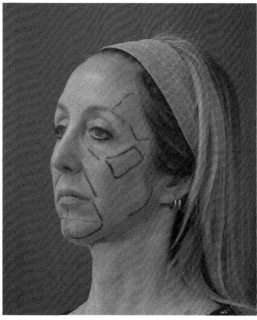

Fig. 1. Preoperative markings.

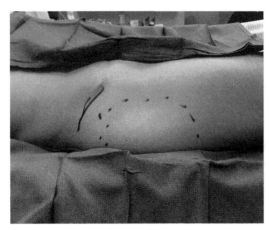

Fig. 2. Lateral thigh harvest site.

with 1-mm side ports. Approximately 40 to 50 mL of aspirate is typically harvested per side using manual suction, assisted by the use of a "Johnnie Lok" to maintain adequate negative pressure. After harvest of the fat, the donor site is closed using a simple Steri-Strip closure of the entry point.

Syringes are allowed to settle by gravity allowing separation of fat from supranatant and infranatant, which are discarded (**Fig. 3**). The 2 syringes now contain microfat given the presence of viable fat cells harvested from small-bore cannulas. Approximately 24 mL of microfat is transferred to 3-mL syringes for the microfat injection (**Fig. 4**). The

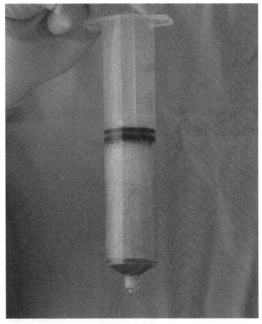

Fig. 3. Harvested microfat before removal of supranatant and infranatant.

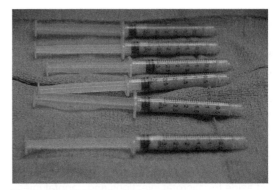

Fig. 4. Microfat ready for injection.

remaining fat is set aside for continued processing into nanofat.

Mechanical processing of nanofat for isolation of AD-MSCs, is performed using the Tulip nanofat system. A set of luer lock connectors is used to emulsify the fat, first with a 2.4-mm luer lock for a total of 40 passes, then a 1.2-mm luer lock for another 40 passes (**Fig. 5**). Any fibrous tissue that obstructs the passage through the luer lock is extracted to prevent clogging of the filter in the following step. The emulsified fat takes on a finer texture and lighter color (**Fig. 6**).

The final step involves a single pass through the nanotransfer filter allowing the final isolation of AD-SVF without surviving adipocytes (**Fig. 7**). This nanofat is also transferred to 3-mL syringes for injection. The nanofat is capable of being injected through small blunt microcannulas (25- or 27-gauge) or 30-gauge needles for superficial intradermal injections.

INJECTION OF MICROFAT

Microfat is injected through 3-mL syringes using a 2-inch 0.7-mm injection cannula. An 18-gauge needle is adequate to create entry points for passage of the 0.7-mm cannula. Injection of microfat proceeds in a top down fashion (**Fig. 8**).

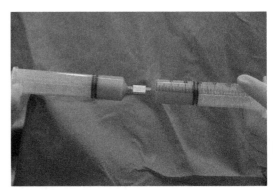

Fig. 5. Luer lock emulsification of fat.

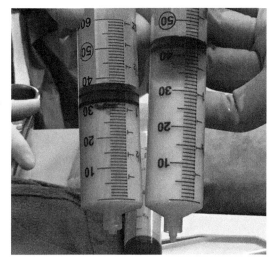

Fig. 6. Comparison of microfat and nanofat.

Approximately 10 to 16 mL of microfat is used per side of the face (total of 20–32 mL of microfat) injected in a deep fashion along the periosteum in all areas except the temple. Care is taken not to overfill these areas to avoid an overfilled or cherubic appearance.

Temple

Temples are addressed with an entry point above the zygomatic arch at the hairline. This allows access to almost the entirety of the temporal fossa from the lateral orbital rim to the superior temporal line and back into the hair-bearing temporal fossa.[24] Approximately 2 to 3 mL of microfat is deposited in small linear aliquots with a fanlike approach and massaged gently.

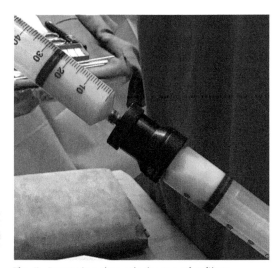

Fig. 7. Processing through the nanofat filter.

Zygomatic Arch and Lateral Cheek

An entry point along the zygoma is used to create a smooth transition from the temple down through the lateral cheek. Approximately 3 mL of microfat is injected into this location, again in small linear aliquots. The injections are performed deep along the periosteum for this injection.

Buccal Space

An entry point lateral to the buccal space allows volumization of the inferior cheek if there is buccal space hollowing. This also helps to improve the transition from the midface to the submalar area. Approximately 1 to 2 mL is used in this region.

Pyriform Aperture

An entry point lateral to the pyriform aperture allows placement of microfat along the periosteum of the lateral and inferior borders of the pyriform aperture.

Chin and Marionette Lines

An entry point is made at the level of the mandibular border anterior to the mandibular ligament and another one more anterior to allow volumization of medial chin. A fanning approach deep along the periosteum is used to volumize this area with a total of 3 to 4 mL per side and in the midline.

Gonial Angle

An entry point superior to the gonial angle allows a fanning technique for volumization of this region. The fingers of the opposite hand are used to guide the inferior extent of the injection to ensure a sharp delineation of the posterior mandible.

INJECTION OF NANOFAT

Nanofat is injected with different techniques depending on the location. For subcutaneous injections, a 25-gauge microcannula is used. A 23-gauge needle is used for creation of the entry points for the microcannula. Use of a smaller cannula is possible; however, the rigidity of the 25-gauge microcannula allows easier injection into the desired areas. For intradermal injections of fine rhytids, a 30-gauge needle is used. Typical volumes of nanofat are 8 to 10 mL per side of the face or a total of 16 to 20 mL (**Fig. 9**).

Upper Face

The glabella, forehead rhytids, and supraorbital/lateral brow region are injected typically with 1 to

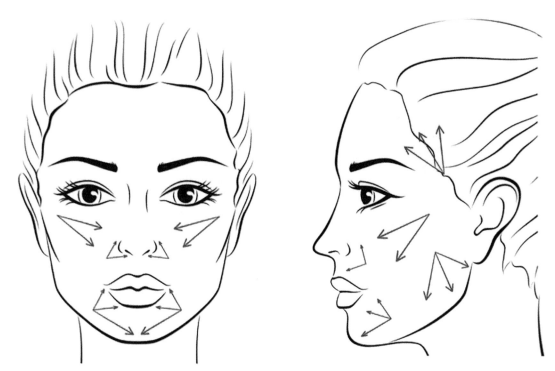

Fig. 8. Location of microfat placement. (*Courtesy of* J. Rihani, MD, FACS, Southlake, TX.)

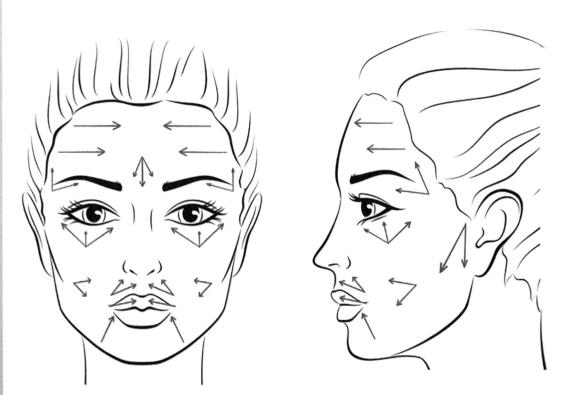

Fig. 9. Location of nanofat placement. (*Courtesy of* J. Rihani, MD, FACS, Southlake, TX.)

2 mL per site using the 25-gauge cannula. The medial upper eyelid can also be addressed, if necessary, in a similar fashion.

Midface

Microcannula injection is used for nanofat placement in the tear trough and lower eyelid, usually in a supraperiosteal location, similar to hyaluronic filler placement. A total of 1 to 2 mL is typically used per side for adequate volumization. If a lower blepharoplasty is simultaneously performed, I typically perform my lower blepharoplasty with fat repositioning before fat injection to avoid movement or suctioning of the nanofat. In this situation, the direction of injections is in a linear, vertical fashion, instead of parallel to the orbital rim (see **Fig. 8**).

Lower Face

The upper lip, nasolabial folds, perioral rhytids, and marionette lines are excellent targets for nanofat injection. A 30-gauge needle is used for subcision and intradermal injection of nanofat into perioral rhytids, allowing a slight wheal to be formed in the skin. Fat injections should be performed carefully using a retrograde threading technique of the cannula to avoid any intravascular complications.

Postoperative Course

Typical swelling and bruising is expected after fat-grafting procedures. Cool compresses are used for the first 3 days and may be accompanied by light facial massage, if not performed in conjunction with another surgical procedure. In areas of intradermal injections or in areas of thin skin, such as the lower eyelid, a slight yellow discoloration can be expected and may persist for a month or 2 following injections, but does resolve. Final volumes are assessed at the 6-month and 1-year time points. Patients are counseled preoperatively that an additional round of fat transfer may be required to achieve desired volumes and optimal correction (**Figs. 10** and **11**).

DISCUSSION

Over the last 30 years, advances in fat grafting have allowed for the fine-tuning of techniques and the art of volumization.[21,25] Volume loss in the face, as we know, does not simply occur through the loss of fat volume, but involves the loss of bone and muscle volume, as well as skin elasticity. These new fat-grafting techniques have decreased the limitations initially seen with traditional fat grafting, while exploring the new frontiers of neocollagenesis for reversing the signs of aging.[26–28]

We are currently in an era of unprecedented popularity of injectable fillers, thanks in part to social media and corporate marketing of HA fillers. Patients and physicians alike now appreciate the role of volume, because it relates to the aging process and facial rejuvenation. Fear of being overfilled, however, is a common concern of many patients who have seen the effect of facial distortion produced by overuse and abuse of many of these synthetic fillers or previously used fat-grafting techniques. As surgeons, however, we

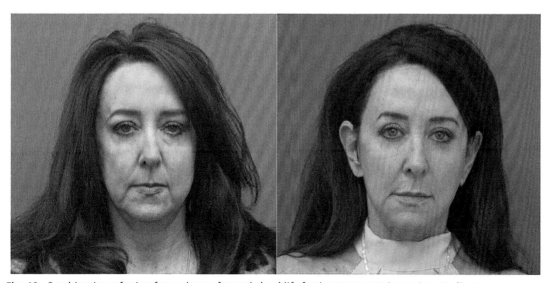

Fig. 10. Combination of microfat and nanofat and cheeklift for improvement in marionette lines.

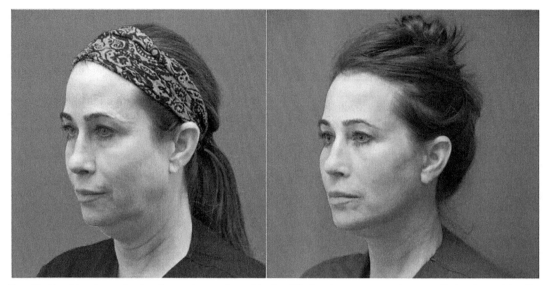

Fig. 11. Combination of microfat and nanofat with facelift for improvement in overall cheek and jawline appearance.

bring a unique perspective that allows for full facial assessment and treatment algorithms that can combine surgical procedures with volume restoration to achieve optimal results.

As knowledge of the role of AD-MSC grows, so do the possibilities of facial rejuvenation. The future holds the ability to not only volumize using fat cells but also to promote new cell and collagen formation through the injection of stromal cells.[29] The promising field of bioregenerative medicine and its applications for facial rejuvenation is still in its early stages and will likely continue to see refinements in the near future. Current techniques that allow for the mechanical isolation of nanofat are simple and easy to perform in either an office or operating room setting, and have been shown to produce viable AD-MSCs as byproducts of the procedure.[17] This has opened the door for new applications of neocollagenesis in patients wanting autologous solutions for facial aging concerns.

Limitations of this procedure include the need for multiple rounds of treatment. Patients are counseled regarding the possibility that a second procedure may be necessary to achieve optimal results and to avoid overfilling during a single treatment. However, given that many patients undergo HA filler treatments annually, I have not found this to be a limitation in my practice. One benefit for patients is the lower cost of fat grafting given the amount of volume afforded by this process without the product cost of the injectable fillers.

Future directions for microfat and nanofat injections include new methods for the efficient harvest of AD-MSCs, standardization of AD-MSC harvest, and expansion of the uses of these products in the clinical setting. For example, one such method was described by Mashiko and colleagues[17] that compared the emulsification technique described here with a "squeeze" technique of cutting adipocytes sharply, which may have reduced the number of damaged mesenchymal stem cells. As clinicians, the idea of expanding the uses of nanofat is quite exciting. One such method is small-volume clinical applications. For example, instead of the larger-volume harvests described, harvesting 10 to 20 mL of nanofat for the improvement in perioral rhytids can also be achieved as an isolated procedure. The results of this procedure have a high patient satisfaction in my practice, with follow-up greater than 2 years.

SUMMARY

The search for the perfect filler remains a long, ongoing one. Facial assessment should begin with an understanding of the changes occurring not only in fat volume but also in muscle and bone volume and skin quality. By using the tools at our disposal, the treating doctor should be able to combine both surgical intervention with volumization to avoid overly pulled or overly filled results. The combination of deeper, structural microfat grafting for volume replacement with more superficial, collagen-forming nanofat provides an optimal solution to produce excellent results.

SURGICAL PEARLS

1. Candidate selection is critical for the procedure. Generally, patients over 40 years of age with adequate donor fat and needing large volumes for replacement of 2 or more regions of the face.
2. Set appropriate patient expectations by discussing the possibility of additional fat transfer sessions at 6 to 12 months.
3. Mark patients preoperatively while sitting upright to avoid the loss of landmarks while they are supine.
4. The lateral thigh is a safe donor site with an adequate fat supply in most women. Abdominal fat may be targeted in men or women without adequate thigh fat.
5. Injections should be performed slowly with small aliquots, injecting only while withdrawing the cannula, to avoid vascular complications.
6. Fat grafting can be combined with other surgical procedures to achieve optimal results.

REFERENCES

1. Peer LA. Loss of weight and volume in human fat grafts. Plast Reconstr Surg 1950;5:217–30.
2. Fournier PF. Facial recontouring with fat grafting. Dermatol Clin 1990;8(3):523–37.
3. American Society for Aesthetic Plastic surgery, procedural Statistics. 2017. Available at: https://www.surgery.org/media/statistics. Accessed September 2018.
4. Pessa JE, Slice DE, Hanz KR, et al. Aging and the shape of the mandible. Plast Reconstr Surg 2008; 121:196–200.
5. Canizares O Jr, Thomson J, Allen R Jr, et al. The effect of processing technique on fat graft survival. Plast Reconstr Surg 2017;140:933–43.
6. Pinski KS, Roenigk HH Jr. Autologous fat transplantation. Long-term follow-up. J Dermatol Surg Oncol 1992;18(3):179–84.
7. Latoni JD, Marshall DM, Wolfe SA. Overgrowth of fat autotransplanted for correction of localized steroid-induced atrophy. Plast Reconstr Surg 2000;106(7): 1566–9.
8. Miller JJ, Popp JC. Fat hypertrophy after autologous fat transfer. Ophthalmic Plast Reconstr Surg 2002; 18(3):228–31.
9. Coleman SR, Lam S, Cohen S, et al. Fat grafting challenges and debates. Atlas Oral Maxillofac Surg Clin North Am 2018;26:81–4.
10. Asken S. Facial liposuction and microlipoinjection. J Dermatol Surg Oncol 1988;14(3):297–305.
11. Tonnard P, Verpaele A, Peeters G, et al. Nanofat grafting: basic research and clinical applications. Plast Reconstr Surg 2013;132(4):1017–26.
12. Lindenblatt N, van Hulle A, Verpaele A, et al. The role of microfat grafting in facial contouring. Aesthet Surg J 2015;35(7):763–71.
13. Bourin P, Bunnell BA, Casteilla L, et al. Stromal cells from the adipose tissue-derived stromal vascular fraction and culture expanded adipose tissue-derived stromal/stem cells: a joint statement of the International Federation for Adipose Therapeutics and Science (IFATS) and the International Society for Cellular Therapy (ISCT). Cytotherapy 2013;15: 641–8.
14. Zuk PA, Zhu M, Ashjian P, et al. Human adipose tissue is a source of multipotent stem cells. Mol Biol Cell 2002;13:4279–95.
15. Zuk PA, Zhu M, Mizuno H, et al. Multilineage cells from human adipose tissue: implications for cell-based therapies. Tissue Eng 2001;7:211–28.
16. Li H, Zimmerlin L, Marra KG, et al. Adipogenic potential of adipose stem cell subpopulations. Plast Reconstr Surg 2011;128:663–72.
17. Mashiko T, Wu SH, Feng J, et al. Mechanical micronization of lipoaspirates: squeeze and emulsification techniques. Plast Reconstr Surg 2017; 139(1):79–90.
18. Eto H, Suga H, Matsumoto D, et al. Characterization of structure and cellular components of aspirated and excised adipose tissue. Plast Reconstr Surg 2009;124(4):1087–97.
19. Harrison BL, Malafa M, Davis K, et al. The discordant histology of grafted fat: a systematic review of the literature. Plast Reconstr Surg 2015;135(3): 542e–55e.
20. Eto H1, Kato H, Suga H, et al. The fate of adipocytes after nonvascularized fat grafting: evidence of early death and replacement of adipocytes. Plast Reconstr Surg 2012;129(5):1081–92.
21. Fournier P. Fat grafting: my technique. Dermatol Surg 2000;26:1117–28.
22. Chaput B, Bertheuil N, Escubes M, et al. Mechanically isolated stromal vascular fraction provides a valid and useful collagenase-free alternative technique: a comparative study. Plast Reconstr Surg 2016;138:807–19.
23. Banyard D, Sarantopoulos C, Brovikova A, et al. Phenotypic analysis of stromal vascular fraction after mechanical shear reveals stress-induced progenitor populations. Plast Reconstr Surg 2016; 138:237e.
24. Rihani J. Aesthetics and rejuvenation of the temple. Facial Plast Surg 2018;34(02):159–63.
25. Marten T, Elyassnia D. Fat grafting in facial rejuvenation. Clin Plast Surg 2015;42:219–52.
26. Wei H, Gu SX, Liang YD, et al. Nanofat-derived stem cells with platelet-rich fibrin improve facial contour remodeling and skin rejuvenation after autologous structural fat transplantation. Oncotarget 2017; 8(No. 40):68542–56.

27. Xu P, Yu Q, Huang H, et al. Nanofat increases dermis thickness and neovascularization in photoaged nude mouse skin. Aesthetic Plast Surg 2018;42:343–51.
28. Uyulmaz S, Macedo NS, Rezaeian F, et al. Nanofat grafting for scar treatment and skin quality improvement. Aesthet Surg J 2018;38(4):421–8.
29. Rigotti G, Charles-de-Sá L, Gontijo-de-Amorim NF, et al. Expanded stem cells, stromal-vascular fraction, and platelet-rich plasma enriched fat: comparing results of different facial rejuvenation approaches in a clinical trial. Aesthet Surg J 2016; 36(3):261–70.

The Benefits of Platelet-Rich Fibrin

Kian Karimi, MD*, Helena Rockwell, BSc

KEYWORDS

- Autologous • Fibrin • Grafting • Platelet • Natural filler • Regenerative therapy • Rejuvenation
- Stem cell

KEY POINTS

- PRF is similar to PRP except that PRF naturally contains fibrin for clot scaffolding and localization of mesenchymal stem cells.
- PRF formation and centrifugation differs from PRP in that there is no anticoagulant and spin times and speeds differ.
- PRF has implied use as a natural filler.
- PRF has had remarked success as a complementary component in surgical and nonsurgical esthetic treatments.
- PRF releases platelet-related therapeutic granules for a longer duration and at a slower rate than PRP.

 Video content accompanies this article at http://www.facialplastic.theclinics.com.

A NEW FRONT IN MEDICAL THERAPIES

Wound healing and tissue regeneration are fundamental goals of medical care. In this context, the use of autologous blood concentrates has emerged. Historically, the primary use of such therapy was in oral maxillofacial surgery;[1] however, its use in surgical and noninvasive esthetic procedures has shown notable success, suggesting a bright future for esthetic and reconstructive medicine.

Autologous platelet therapy gained popularity in the 1990s with the use of platelet-rich plasma (PRP), which has since found several medical applications. The focus of this article is the next generation of autologous blood concentrate therapy, platelet-rich fibrin (PRF), and its roles in esthetic medicine. The significance of these developments will become apparent throughout the review of the composition of whole blood.

WHOLE BLOOD COMPOSITION

Blood is composed of plasma (55%) and cells (45%).[2] Plasma consists mostly of water (92%), as well as soluble proteins, electrolytes, and metabolic wastes. The most notable soluble constituent is fibrinogen, a clotting protein. When tissue and vascular injury occur, thrombin enzymatically converts fibrinogen to insoluble fibrin.[2–5] Fibrin then acts as the binding scaffold for platelets and erythrocytes in clot formation, which is the essential first step in wound healing and tissue regeneration.[1–4] Beyond plasma, red blood cells (erythrocytes), white blood cells (leukocytes), and platelets (thrombocytes) constitute the remaining cellular component of whole blood.[2] Erythrocytes are the most abundant, comprising about 44% of total blood composition, whereas leukocytes and thrombocytes constitute the buffy coat at less than 1%.[2]

Disclosure Statement: Dr K. Karimi is the medical director of CosmoFrance, which manufactures and distributes PRF centrifuges and tubes. H. Rockwell has nothing to disclose.
Rejuva Medical Aesthetics, 11645 Wilshire Boulevard, Suite 605, Los Angeles, CA 90025, USA
* Corresponding author.
E-mail address: kiankarimi@gmail.com

Facial Plast Surg Clin N Am 27 (2019) 331–340
https://doi.org/10.1016/j.fsc.2019.03.005
1064-7406/19/© 2019 Elsevier Inc. All rights reserved.

Centrifuging whole blood conveniently separates its components according to density. Erythrocytes collect at the bottom of the tube, forming the hematocrit layer; the thin, white-tinted buffy coat settles at the top of the erythrocytes; and plasma forms the supernatant.[1,2,6] Varying centrifugation speed and duration further separates blood concentrate components. Anticoagulants or enzymatic supplements may be required to separate PRP and platelet-poor plasma (PPP),[1,7] the former with enough platelets for therapeutic use, yet less abundant than PPP at roughly 25% and 75% of the supernatant volume, respectively.[8]

WHAT IS AUTOLOGOUS BLOOD CONCENTRATE THERAPY?
First, There Was PRP

The widely accepted mechanism of PRP therapy is growth factor secretion from platelet alpha granules. When activated in vivo through injury and clot formation, alpha factors bind to the platelet surface and release platelet-derived growth factors, transforming growth factors, fibroblastic growth factor, epithelial cell growth factor, insulin-like growth factor, and vascular endothelial growth factor (**Table 1**).[1,8–10] Collectively, these signals

help stimulate mesenchymal stem cell (MSC) migration and differentiation at the site of clot formation.[1,11,12] For PRP, induced clot formation localizes growth factor secretion to its implemented site.[1,13]

In aging skin, PRP's targeted growth factor secretion promotes fibroblast proliferation and gene expression that stimulates type I collagenesis.[14] To harness these abilities, PRP must first be produced using anticoagulant.[6,10] Second, to ensure that platelet activation and fibrin clot formation occurs, calcium chloride and thrombin, which is often bovine derived,[6] must be added to the PRP preparation[6,9,10,13,15]; using bovine-derived thrombin poses the risk of inducing adverse immunologic reactions.[6,16] Alternatively, additives can be omitted and trust that activation and clot formation occur spontaneously in vivo,[13] which is not guaranteed. If PRP's production process potentially compromises its benefits, then its antiaging properties may also be at risk. Fortunately, PRF is a readily available promising alternative.

The Next Generation of Autologous Platelet Therapy: Platelet Rich Fibrin

PRF was first introduced in 2000 by Joseph Choukroun and colleagues.[17] PRF offers all the clinical benefits of PRP as well as a naturally forming fibrin scaffold that guides clot formation, serves as a supportive template for tissue regeneration, and that sustains growth factors and stem cells.[6,10,18]

In contrast to PRP, PRF is obtained by centrifuging whole blood without any additives.[10,15] Without anticoagulant, PRF spontaneously forms a fibrin matrix gelatinous clot[9,10,15] that confines growth factor secretion to the clotting site. In tissue repair, recruited fibroblasts reorganize this fibrin matrix and initiate collagen synthesis.[19] Thus, the combined effects of growth factor secretion and fibroblast recruitment in PRF work synergistically to promote collagenesis and tissue regeneration.

Injury-induced growth factor signaling recruits MSCs to the compromised site[11,12,20,21] where they subsequently differentiate.[11,18,21] Surgeries and injections simulate local injury and trigger the same signaling cascade. Applying PRF with these treatments localizes and enhances the regenerative processes spurred by the body's natural response to injury. In the context of attracting, entrapping, and sustaining MSCs, research has also revealed that fibrin serves as a successful culture medium and carrier of MSCs,[18,22,23] which preserves the paracrine functions essential in conferring their regenerative effects.[24]

Table 1	
Platelet therapy growth factor functions	
Platelet-derived growth factor (PDGFaa, PDGFbb, PDGFab)	• Triggers the activities of neutrophils, fibroblasts, and macrophages • Chemoattractant/cell proliferator • Stimulates mesenchymal cell lineages
Transforming growth factor (TGFβ1, TGFβ2, TGFβ3)	• Promotes cellular differentiation and replication • Stimulates matrix and collagen synthesis • Stimulates fibroblast activity and collagen production
Vascular endothelial growth factor (VEGF)	• Angiogenesis • Stimulates synthesis of basal lamina
Fibroblastic growth factor (FGF)	• Angiogenesis • Fibroblast production
Epithelial cell growth factor (ECGF)	• Stimulates epithelial cell replication
Insulin-like growth factor (IGF-1)	• Promotes cellular growth and proliferation

PRF also sustains other vital cells, including leukocytes.[18] Analyzing the cellular content of the PRF clot reveals that most leukocytes within a whole-blood sample are contained within PRF after centrifugation.[10,25] These leukocytes secrete signaling factors that further stimulate tissue repair[1,26] and MSC recruitment.[12]

MSCs bear important regenerative applications; their multipotency allows them to give rise to several tissues including bone, cartilage, adipose, dermis, and other mesodermal tissues.[27–29] MSCs in peripheral blood have been isolated[30,31] and shown to proliferate and differentiate on stimulation.[21,32] Di Liddo and colleagues[33] detected in vitro multipotent stem cell markers within PRF, and reported that a fraction of cells in PRF express defining phenotypic features of MSCs. Therefore, PRF establishes a local environment conducive to MSC migration and may also serve as a stem cell source.

Altering centrifugation duration and speed allows for manipulation of product volume and clotting onset. Broadly, this yields 2 categories of PRF:

1. Injectable PRF: clot formation occurs around 15 minutes postcentrifugation[34]

2. PRF that coagulates during centrifugation: this is most useful when a biological membrane or a physiologic glue is needed (**Fig. 1**)

Platelet-Rich Plasma Versus Platelet Rich Fibrin

PRF has various advantages over PRP. With PRP and other past-generation platelet concentrates, growth factor release is initially rapid, yielding short-lived, early healing benefits without long-term improvement.[15] The relatively short half-lives of growth factors,[13,35] in conjunction with their abundant and rapid release following PRP activation,[36] supports this lack of prolonged efficacy, because tissue receptor saturation may prevent additional growth factors from binding a receptor before their degradation.[13] Recall that preparing functional PRP requires external additives, which brings uncertainty about its spontaneous activation in vivo. Thus, functional PRP is either nonautologous, or its efficacy is unguaranteed.

Contrastingly, PRF requires no additives. Activation and fibrin clot formation are based on known, intrinsic properties of blood, and the timeliness of activation is relatively well understood.

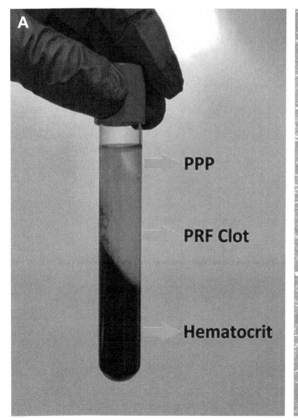
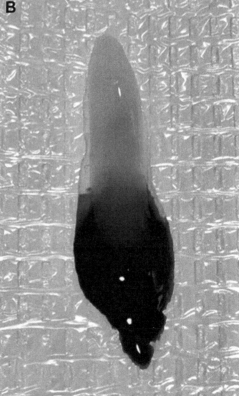

PPP

PRF Clot

Hematocrit

Fig. 1. (*A*) Visualization of the resulting blood concentrate layers from centrifugation to immediately procure a PRF clot. (*B*) The PRF clot removed from the centrifuge tube.

Furthermore, the holistically autologous nature of PRF reduces the risk of immunogenic reaction and disease transmission.[6]

Most notably, in comparison with PRP's rapid growth factor release, PRF releases growth factors for an extended duration of time: up to 7 days for most growth factors,[15] and even longer for others.[37] It is proposed that PRF's composition aids in preventing rapid proteolysis of growth factors,[38] thereby enabling prolonged secretion. In addition, the slow polymerization and remodeling of the fibrin matrix within PRF, compared with PRP's more rapid, haphazard polymerization, effectively sustains growth factors and other critical cells.[7,9,15] Masuki and colleagues[39] concluded from their comparative analysis that growth factor concentrations are generally higher in PRF than PRP, a finding that supports PRF's marked efficacy in stimulating angiogenesis, wound healing, and tissue regeneration. As previously mentioned, growth factors chemotactically attract MSCs. Therefore, it is reasonably assumed that PRF's sustained growth factor secretion, in comparison with PRP, more strongly induces MSC migration to the site of its application, a conclusion that is further backed by comparative in vitro studies.[37,40]

Beyond their chemotactic and compositional differences, PRF and PRP undergo different centrifugation premises for their procurement (**Fig. 2**). The low-speed centrifugation of PRF tends to better preserve the beneficial cellular content within the resulting PRF layer,[26,34,41] whereas high-speed centrifugation, such as that seen in the hardspin stage of PRP preparation,[10] tends to push most cells to the bottom of the tube.[26]

Regarding cost, PRP incurs the cost of separating gel, anticoagulant, and activation additives, whereas PRF does not. PRF use implies reduced costs for provider and patient alike.

APPLICATIONS OF PLATELET RICH FIBRIN

The following text outlines a few of the many applications of PRF in cosmetic medicine and surgery. Other applications not discussed, but worth mentioning, include enhanced healing following ablative skin resurfacing laser treatments and collagen induction with microneedling.

Natural Filler

Aging skin naturally loses collagen, elasticity, and volume. The dermis thins and the fibroblast

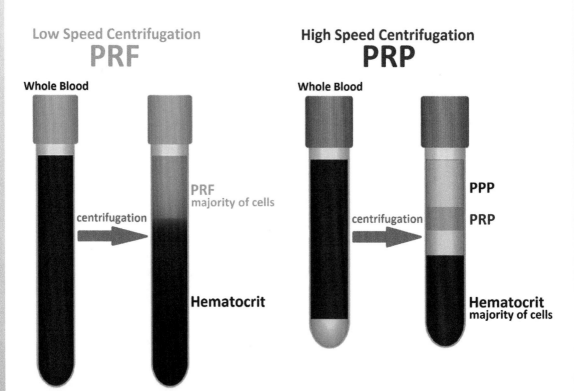

Fig. 2. Separations achieved by each blood concentrates' respective centrifugation parameters. The white separating gel and anticoagulant necessary for preparing PRP is visualized at the bottom of the whole blood tube and is pictured separating PRP and the hematocrit in the PRP postcentrifugation tube. (*Courtesy of* CosmoFrance, Inc., Miami, FL.)

population declines, reducing the production of collagen and hyaluronic acid.[42] As collagen decreases by approximately 1% yearly,[43] skin laxity and wrinkling become apparent.[14,43] Our skin also loses moisture because the hydrophilic hyaluronic acid concentration declines.[44] Consequently, the dermis loses turgidity,[45] resulting in volume loss and unesthetic changes. Stimulating collagenesis and hyaluronic acid content within aging skin may overcome these changes. Here, PRF shows promise.

With high concentrations and slow release of fibroblastic growth factors, PRF, when injected beneath the skin, should stimulate fibroblast formation and subsequently increase collagen and hyaluronic acid content. PRF also enmeshes hyaluronic acid, sustaining it where injected.[7] As it forms a gel, PRF produces an immediate volumization effect; although this volumization lasts only a few weeks, repeated treatments yield long-term effects from prolonged collagen production and localized regenerative activity.

In his own practice, the primary author has found success with injecting PRF alone as a natural, autologous dermal filler, which has resulted in volume restoration of hollowing tear troughs, improved fine lines, and homogenization of pigmentation irregularities with repeat treatments (**Fig. 3**).

The author has also treated patients with a combination of PRF and hyaluronic acid filler (**Fig. 4**, Video 1). Together, PRF and filler synergistically improve moisture retention and create a scaffold for collagen growth as the body metabolizes the filler over time. The author has anecdotally found that a concentration of 2 parts filler to 1 part PRF will lead to a sustained filler effect and still harness the advantages of the PRF.

Fat Grafting

Autologous fat transfer, although slightly more invasive than office-based hyaluronic acid fillers, efficaciously restores volume loss. Unlike conventional dermal fillers, fat grafts provide potentially permanent volume restoration; however, only roughly half of the transferred cells survive.[46] Fortunately, PRF shows promise in improving fat retention (**Fig. 5**).

Adipose tissue is considered an exceptional stem cell source.[28] Furthermore, subcutaneous fat is an especially attractive source of progenitor cells because of its accessibility, abundance, and the existence of a supportive stromal vascular fraction (SVF).[47] The SVF of the abdominal subcutaneous tissues is regarded as an exceptional fat harvesting location considering its abundant supply of adipose-derived stem cells.[47] However, stem cell viability can be difficult to sufficiently sustain while in transit during fat transfer. Liu and colleagues[48] highlighted the enhancement of fat transfer with PRF supplementation, detailing that implementing PRF reduced resorption and improved retention of fat grafts. PRF's effect on fat survival likely results from its prolonged growth

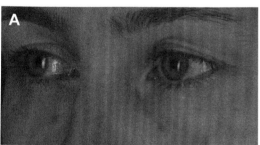
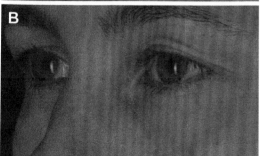

Fig. 3. A 45-year-old female patient (*A*) before and (*B*) after 3 treatments of infraorbital PRF injections spaced 4 to 6 weeks apart to correct pigmentation irregularities, stimulate volume restoration, improve fine lines, and reduce under-eye hollowing.

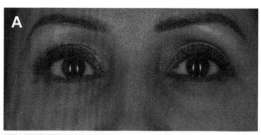
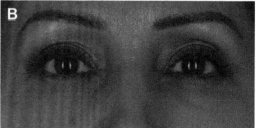

Fig. 4. (*A*) Before and (*B*) immediately after treatment of a 40-year-old female patient with hyaluronic acid filler and PRF injected to infraorbital hollows.

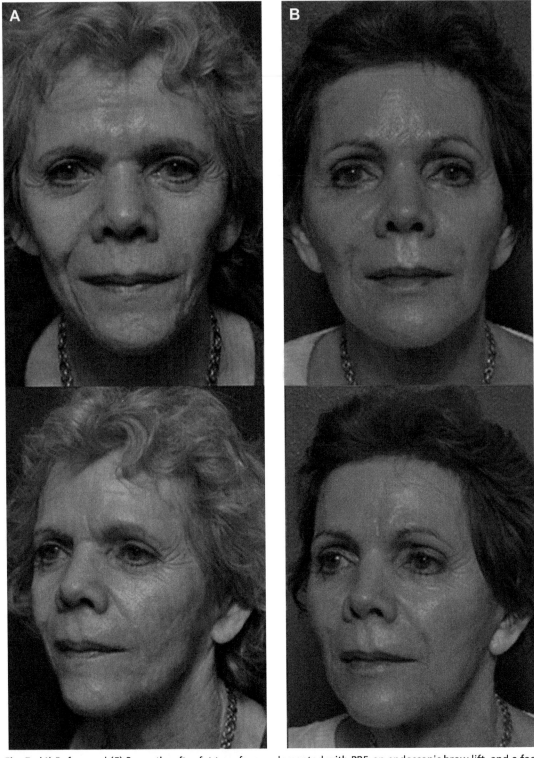

Fig. 5. (*A*) Before and (*B*) 3 months after fat transfer supplemented with PRF, an endoscopic brow lift, and a face lift were performed on this 66-year-old female patient.

factor release and the ability of the autologous fibrin matrix to sufficiently support stem cell transfer. A study by Keyhan and colleagues[49] supported this premise, reporting that PRF more effectively improved fat graft retention than PRP. Video 2 depicts the process conducted to supplement fat transfer with PRF.

Facial Surgery

As invasive treatments, facial surgeries elicit strong clotting and wound-healing responses.

The resulting blood clots consist mainly of erythrocytes.[1] Applying PRF to the surgical site effectively replaces the abundance of erythrocytes with fibrin, leukocytes, stem cells, and platelet-derived growth factors. This results in accelerated wound healing and attraction of MSCs to the site, laying the foundation for tissue regeneration, collagen remodeling, and a sustained cosmetic result.

In rhinoplasties, cartilage grafts are frequently needed to achieve optimal results. Cartilage grafts are formed from diced autologous or cadaver

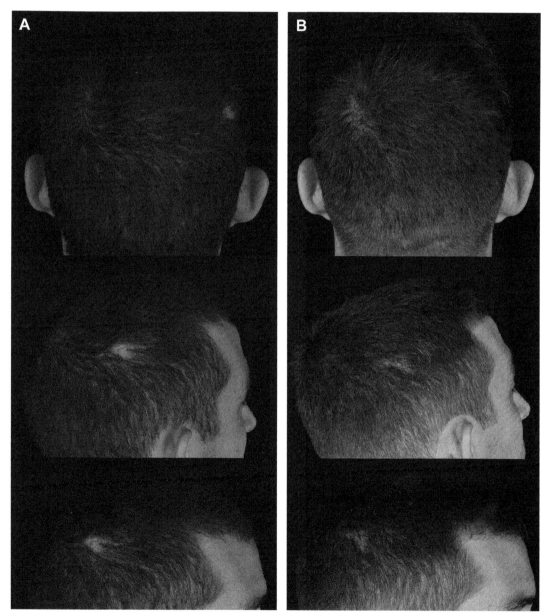

Fig. 6. (*A*) Before and (*B*) after 1 session of PRF injections to treat the appearance and hair growth of a lateral parietal trauma-induced scar of a 28-year-old male patient. Progress photos were obtained 6 months after treatment. Before treatment, hair growth was dormant for 5 weeks.

cartilage. When used alone, diced cartilage may scatter after placement, resulting in palpable or visible structural irregularities.[50,51] PRF aids in forming and depositing cartilage grafts by acting as a physiologic glue that enhances the consistency and pliability of the grafts and reduces the probability of graft rejection owing to its autologous nature (Video 3). Studied in a rabbit model, PRF effectively improved cartilage graft viability,[50] and, in another study, it stimulated cartilage regeneration more so than PRP.[34]

Hair Loss and Scar Therapy

The primary author has found that PRF injections improve scar appearance and stimulate hair growth where hair follicles are present but inactive (**Fig. 6**).

THE FUTURE OF PLATELET RICH FIBRIN

The widespread applications of PRF solidify its place among autologous blood concentrate therapies as both a primary and supplementary medical tool. Further research is expected to uncover additional benefits to be obtained from PRF's bioavailability, autologous nature, and regenerative properties.

SUPPLEMENTARY DATA

Supplementary data related to this article can be found online at https://doi.org/10.1016/j.fsc.2019.03.005.

ACKNOWLEDGMENTS

The authors thank Marissa Kudo for her additions in assembly of information for this article, and Fred Wilson for his editorial contributions.

REFERENCES

1. Garg AK. Autologous blood concentrates. Batavia (IL): Quintessence Publishing Co. Inc.; 2018.
2. Mescher AL. Blood. In: Junqueira's basic histology text & atlas. 15th edition. New York: McGraw-Hill; 2013. Chapter 12.
3. Brummel KE, Butenas S, Mann KG. An integrated study of fibrinogen during blood coagulation. J Biol Chem 1999;274(32):22862–70.
4. Mann KG, Brummel K, Butenas S. What is all that thrombin for? J Thromb Haemost 2003;1(7):1504–14.
5. Undas A, Ariëns RA. Fibrin clot structure and function. Arterioscler Thromb Vasc Biol 2011;31(12):88–99.
6. Utomo DN, Mahyudin F, Hernugrahanto KD, et al. Implantation of platelet rich fibrin and allogenic mesenchymal stem cells facilitate the healing of muscle injury: an experimental study on animal. Int J Surg Open 2018;11:4–9.
7. Dohan DM, Choukroun J, Diss A, et al. Platelet-rich fibrin (PRF): a second-generation platelet concentrate. Part II: platelet-related biologic features. Oral Surg Oral Med Oral Pathol Oral Radiol Endod 2006; 101(3):45–50.
8. Marx RE, Carlson ER, Eichstaedt RM, et al. Platelet-rich plasma: growth factor enhancement for bone grafts. Oral Surg Oral Med Oral Pathol Oral Radiol Endod 1998;85(6):638–46.
9. Dohan DM, Choukroun J, Diss A, et al. Platelet-rich fibrin (PRF): a second-generation platelet concentrate. Part I: technological concepts and evolution. Oral Surg Oral Med Oral Pathol Oral Radiol Endod 2006;101(3):37–44.
10. Ehrenfest DMD, Rasmusson L, Albrektsson T. Classification of platelet concentrates: from pure platelet-rich plasma (P-PRP) to leucocyte- and platelet-rich fibrin (L-PRF). Trends Biotechnol 2009; 27(3):158–67.
11. Boer HD, Verseyden C, Ulfman L, et al. Fibrin and activated platelets cooperatively guide stem cells to a vascular injury and promote differentiation towards an endothelial cell phenotype. Arterioscler Thromb Vasc Biol 2006;26(7):1653–9.
12. Ponte AL, Marais E, Gallay N, et al. The in vitro migration capacity of human bone marrow mesenchymal stem cells: comparison of chemokine and growth factor chemotactic activities. Stem Cells 2007;25(7):1737–45.
13. Cavallo C, Roffi A, Grigolo B, et al. Platelet-rich plasma: the choice of activation method affects the release of bioactive molecules. Biomed Res Int 2016;2016:1–7.
14. Kim DH, Je YJ, Kim CD, et al. Can platelet-rich plasma be used for skin rejuvenation? Evaluation of effects of platelet-rich plasma on human dermal fibroblast. Ann Dermatol 2011;23(4):424–31.
15. Ehrenfest DMD, Peppo GMD, Doglioli P, et al. Slow release of growth factors and thrombospondin-1 in Choukrouns platelet-rich fibrin (PRF): a gold standard to achieve for all surgical platelet concentrates technologies. Growth Factors 2009;27(1):63–9.
16. Raja VS, Naidu EM. Platelet-rich fibrin: evolution of a second-generation platelet concentrate. Indian J Dent Res 2008;19(1):42–6.
17. Choukroun J, Adda F, Schoeffer C, et al. PRF: an opportunity in perio-implantology. Implantodontie 2000; 42:55–62.
18. Choukroun J, Diss A, Simonpieri A, et al. Platelet-rich fibrin (PRF): a second-generation platelet concentrate. Part IV: clinical effects on tissue healing. Oral Surg Oral Med Oral Pathol Oral Radiol Endod 2006;101(3):56–60.
19. Tuan T-L, Song A, Chang S, et al. In Vitro Fibroplasia: matrix contraction, cell growth, and collagen production of

fibroblasts cultured in fibrin gels. Exp Cell Res 1996; 223(1):127–34.

20. Badiavas EV, Abedi M, Butmarc J, et al. Participation of bone marrow derived cells in cutaneous wound healing. J Cell Physiol 2003;196(2):245–50.

21. Xu L, Li G. Circulating mesenchymal stem cells and their clinical implications. J Orthop Translat 2014; 2(1):1–7.

22. Bensaïd W, Triffitt J, Blanchat C, et al. A biodegradable fibrin scaffold for mesenchymal stem cell transplantation. Biomaterials 2003;24(14):2497–502.

23. Catelas I, Sese N, Wu BM, et al. Human mesenchymal stem cell proliferation and osteogenic differentiation in fibrin gels in vitro. Tissue Eng 2006;12(8): 2385–96.

24. Kim I, Lee SK, Yoon JI, et al. Fibrin glue improves the therapeutic effect of MSCs by sustaining survival and paracrine function. Tissue Eng Part A 2013; 19(21–22):2373–81.

25. Ehrenfest DMD, Corso MD, Diss A, et al. Three-dimensional architecture and cell composition of a Choukrouns platelet-rich fibrin clot and membrane. J Periodontol 2010;81(4):546–55.

26. Ghanaati S, Booms P, Orlowska A, et al. Advanced platelet-rich fibrin: a new concept for cell-based tissue engineering by means of inflammatory cells. J Oral Implantol 2014;40(6):679–89.

27. Kim N, Cho S-G. Clinical applications of mesenchymal stem cells. Korean J Intern Med 2013; 28(4):387–402.

28. Kobolak J, Dinnyes A, Memic A, et al. Mesenchymal stem cells: identification, phenotypic characterization, biological properties and potential for regenerative medicine through biomaterial micro-engineering of their niche. Methods 2016;99:62–8.

29. Caplan AI. Mesenchymal stem cells. J Orthop Res 1991;9(5):641–50.

30. Rochefort GY, Delorme B, Lopez A, et al. Multipotential mesenchymal stem cells are mobilized into peripheral blood by hypoxia. Stem Cells 2006;24(10): 2202–8.

31. Tondreau T, Meuleman N, Delforge A, et al. Mesenchymal stem cells derived from CD133-positive cells in mobilized peripheral blood and cord blood: proliferation, Oct4 expression, and plasticity. Stem Cells 2005;23:1105–12.

32. Chong P-P, Selvaratnam L, Abbas AA, et al. Human peripheral blood derived mesenchymal stem cells demonstrate similar characteristics and chondrogenic differentiation potential to bone marrow derived mesenchymal stem cells. J Orthop Res 2011;30(4):634–42.

33. Di Liddo R, Bertalot T, Borean A, et al. Leucocyte and platelet-rich fibrin: a carrier of autologous multipotent cells for regenerative medicine. J Cell Mol Med 2018;22(3):1840–54.

34. Raouf MAE, Wang X, Miusi S, et al. Injectable-platelet rich fibrin using the low speed centrifugation concept improves cartilage regeneration when compared to platelet-rich plasma. Platelets 2017;1–9. https://doi.org/10.1080/09537104.2017.1401058.

35. Creaney L, Hamilton B. Growth factor delivery methods in the management of sports injuries: the state of play. Br J Sports Med 2008;42:314–20.

36. Kobayashi E, Flückiger L, Fujioka-Kobayashi M, et al. Comparative release of growth factors from PRP, PRF, and advanced-PRF. Clin Oral Investig 2016;20(9):2353–60.

37. He L, Lin Y, Hu X, et al. A comparative study of platelet-rich fibrin (PRF) and platelet-rich plasma (PRP) on the effect of proliferation and differentiation of rat osteoblasts in vitro. Oral Surg Oral Med Oral Pathol Oral Radiol Endod 2009;108:707–13.

38. Lundquist R, Dziegiel MH, Ågren MS. Bioactivity and stability of endogenous fibrogenic factors in platelet-rich fibrin. Wound Repair Regen 2008; 16(3):356–63.

39. Masuki H, Okudera T, Watanebe T, et al. Growth factor and pro-inflammatory cytokine contents in platelet-rich plasma (PRP), plasma rich in growth factors (PRGF), advanced platelet-rich fibrin (A-PRF), and concentrated growth factors (CGF). Int J Implant Dent 2016;2(1):1–6.

40. Schär MO, Diaz-Romero J, Kohl S, et al. Platelet-rich concentrates differentially release growth factors and induce cell migration in vitro. Clin Orthop Relat Res 2015;473(5):1635–43.

41. Fujioka-Kobayashi M, Miron RJ, Hernandez M, et al. Optimized platelet-rich fibrin with the low-speed concept: growth factor release, biocompatibility, and cellular response. J Periodontol 2017;88(1):112–21.

42. Farage MA, Miller KW, Elsner P, et al. Characteristics of the aging skin. Adv Wound Care 2013;2(1): 5–10.

43. Ganceviciene R, Liakou AI, Theodoridis A, et al. Skin anti-aging strategies. Dermatoendocrinol 2012;4(3): 308–19.

44. Papakonstantinou E, Roth M, Karakiulakis G. Hyaluronic acid: a key molecule in skin aging. Dermatoendocrinol 2012;4(3):253–8.

45. Ghersetich I, Lolli T, Campanile G, et al. Hyaluronic acid in cutaneous intrinsic aging. Int J Dermatol 1994;33(2):119–22.

46. Peer LA. Loss of weight and volume in human fat grafts. Plast Reconstr Surg 1950;5(3):217–30.

47. Jurgens WJFM, Oedayrajsingh-Varma MJ, Helder MN, et al. Effect of tissue-harvesting site on yield of stem cells derived from adipose tissue: implications for cell-based therapies. Cell Tissue Res 2008;332(3): 415–26.

48. Liu B, Tan X-Y, Liu Y-P, et al. The adjuvant use of stromal vascular fraction and platelet-rich fibrin for

autologous adipose tissue transplantation. Tissue Eng Part C Methods 2013;19(1):1–14.

49. Keyhan SO, Hemmat S, Badri AA, et al. Use of platelet-rich fibrin and platelet-rich plasma in combination with fat graft: which is more effective during facial lipostructure? J Oral Maxillofac Surg 2013; 71(3):610–21.

50. Göral A, Aslan C, Küçükzeybek BB, et al. Platelet-rich fibrin improves the viability of diced cartilage grafts in a rabbit model. Aesthet Surg J 2016; 36(4):153–62.

51. Daniel RK, Calvert JW. Diced cartilage grafts in rhinoplasty surgery. Plast Reconstr Surg 2004;113(7): 2156–71.

Silhouette Instalift
Benefits to a Facial Plastic Surgery Practice

Kaete A. Archer, MD[a],*, Roberto Eloy Garcia, MD[b]

KEYWORDS

- Silhouette instalift • Thread lift • Nonsurgical • Instalift

KEY POINTS

- The Silhouette Instalift has an improved safety and efficacy profile over barbed suture thread lifting.
- Silhouette Instalift sutures lift and reposition the midfacial tissues.
- Silhouette Instalift sutures have immediate results with minimal downtime.

INTRODUCTION

Today's facial plastic surgeon offers many procedures to rejuvenate the aging face and neck. Surgical and nonsurgical procedures are chosen not only based on training and experience but also safety, efficacy, cost, anatomic findings, goals, expectations, and lifestyle. As the market for facial plastic surgery expands to a younger generation of patients, and as more patients become wary of potential risks and complications of surgery, there has been an increased interest in minimally invasive procedures with minimal downtime and maximal results. Traditionally, these patients are in their late 40s to 50s, have a busy lifestyle, and are not interested in 2 weeks of downtime. These patients are interested in the "latest and greatest" with an affinity for technology and may have considered a "weekend facelift."

This shift is evident in the data for surgical versus nonsurgical facial rejuvenation released by the American Society for Aesthetic Plastic Surgery (ASAPS). According to ASAPS, between 1997 and 2016, surgical facial rejuvenation saw a 19.5% increase, while nonsurgical facial rejuvenation saw a 6956.6% increase.[1] This has led to a continued search for less-invasive methods to improve facial aging, particularly skin ptosis.

Suture procedures were first described in the 1980s, when nonabsorbable polypropylene threads became available. In 1999, Sulamanidze obtained worldwide patents for the subdermal "Aptos" thread product. The technique of barbed suture lift was subsequently published by Sulamanidze and colleagues[2] in December 2001, with a formal series presented in 2002.[3] Variations of this technique included Contour Thread, also referred to as Thread Lift or (with a looped suture) Loop Lift (Surgical Specialties, Corp, Reading, PA), and the Aptos lift or Feather lift (Kolster Methods, Inc, Anaheim, CA).

Both suture design and treatment have evolved. The original Aptos suture was a multiple-dented suture for additional traction on tissue. This design was modified to be bidirectional, with the barbs oriented so that tissue would be retained in the central region of the suture without the need for anchoring at either end. It was then redesigned as a multiple-barbed polypropylene suture intended to provide traction and suspension unidirectionally.

Disclosure Statement: The authors have no commercial or financial conflicts of interest and no funding sources to disclose.
^a Private Practice, Aesthetic Institute of Manhattan for Facial and Plastic Surgery, 460 Park Avenue, 17th Floor, New York, NY 10022, USA; ^b Private Practice, Contoura Facial Plastic Surgery, 190 Florida A1A North Suite 1, Ponte Vedra Beach, FL 32082, USA
* Corresponding author.
E-mail address: drarcher@aestheticinstituteofmanhattan.com

In 2004, the US Food and Drug Administration (FDA) approved unidirectional barbed thread lifting (Contour Lift, Aptos Lift) for mid and lower facial rejuvenation.[4,5] These sutures were permanent, polypropylene, barbed sutures intended to catch and lift the dermis in a unidirectional fashion, allowing for fixation of the skin and, to a lesser extent, the soft tissue in an elevated position.[6–9] Despite their revolutionary approach, these barbed sutures caused many complications. Patients had severe pain, skin dimpling, and foreign body reactions.[10–13] Cutting the suture to create the barbs left the overall suture weakened, leading to breakage and decreased longevity (3–6 months).[14] Because these sutures were permanent, infection and extrusion were common. Because of the barbed nature, they were difficult to remove.

Contour Lift lost FDA approval in 2007 a result of serious complications.[15] In 2009, a retrospective review of 33 face and neck rejuvenation cases using nonabsorbable suspension sutures concluded that the use of this treatment could not be justified based on the high number of reported adverse events and complications, including thread breakage and extrusion, skin dimpling, superficial hemorrhages, mild asymmetry, ecchymosis, erythema, edema, inflammation, persistent pain, and poor long-term sustainability of the suture.[16]

More recently, the cosmetic market has been reintroduced to "thread lifting" with completely absorbable, advanced suspension technology for suspending facial tissue and restoring facial volume. Silhouette Soft (Sinclair Pharma, London, UK) is a family of fully resorbable, bidirectional, cone-based, self-anchoring suspension sutures made of poly-L-lactic acid (PLLA) with injection molded cones made of polylactide/glycolide (PLGA) affixed to the suture. Silhouette Soft was introduced to the European market as a Class III Medical Device in 2012 for midface improvement by Silhouette Lift, Inc.[17,18] Silhouette Lift, Inc was acquired by Sinclair Pharma in 2014.[15]

In April 2015, the FDA-approved Silhouette Instalift absorbable suture suspension for the on-label indication of midface suspension to lift, recontour, and reposition midfacial subdermal tissues.[15,19] The company introduced the Silhouette Instalift procedure to US markets in 2016 based on the success of the Silhouette Soft, also making this suture with knots and cones fully absorbable and fully biodegradable using PLLA and PLGA.[15] Unlike the Silhouette Soft sutures, the entire Silhouette Instalift suture of knots and cones is the combination of 82% PLLA and 18% PLGA. Silhouette Instalift was initially approved with a permanent suspension suture anchored to the temporalis fascia. In June 2017, the FDA revised the indication to remove the absolute need for permanent, open suture fixation.[15]

Indications for the Silhouette Instalift procedure include signs of moderate midfacial tissue descent—nasolabial folds, downturned oral commissures, and marionette folds (Figs. 1–4). Advantages of the procedure include minimal downtime of 1 day without makeup, a natural appearance, and immediate results. The procedure is done under local anesthesia. Start-to-finish including set up and anesthesia takes about 45 to 60 minutes. The results last about 18–36 months and can be performed in combination with other nonsurgical modalities for overall rejuvenation.[20,21]

The PLLA/PLGA suspension sutures have good tensile strength and their design assures a large surface area to enhance tissue integration.[22] A fully absorbable product reduces the risk of infection or need for removal. By using biodegradable cones, instead of barbs, the structural integrity of suture is kept intact along with a decreased risk of dimpling, extrusion, and palpability.[23] Silhouette sutures do not rely on anchoring of the dermis like their barbed predecessor, but rather on capturing the retaining ligament anatomy and lifting the facial compartments in a parachute fashion. This absorbable suture helps to recreate a youthful facial shape by not only lifting ptotic tissue, but also increasing collagen production in the midface area, which is explored in more detail below.[21]

SILHOUETTE INSTALIFT SUTURE DESIGN AND MATERIAL

The Silhouette Instalift sutures are a combination of knots and cones with 23-gauge straight, stainless-steel needles preattached on both ends. The needles are 12 cm long with a 5-mm depth marker to aid insertion of the needles into the tissue. The sutures are designed with 8, 12, or 16 cones. An equal number of cones are positioned on each side of a 2-cm cone-free central zone. The 8 cone sutures are recommended for midface suspension. Each set of cones faces the opposite direction, pointing toward the end of the suture, hence the term "bidirectional" (Fig. 5). Each cone is separated by "hand-tied" knots that require tightening before suture placement. The cones are evenly spaced and designed to decrease risk of migration and extrusion. The entire 8-cone suture is 30 cm long.

The sutures are supplied in a pack of 2. All products are supplied sterile (ethylene oxide) for single use only.[18] The sutures should be stored between 0°C and 8°C in a dry place, out of direct sunlight.[18]

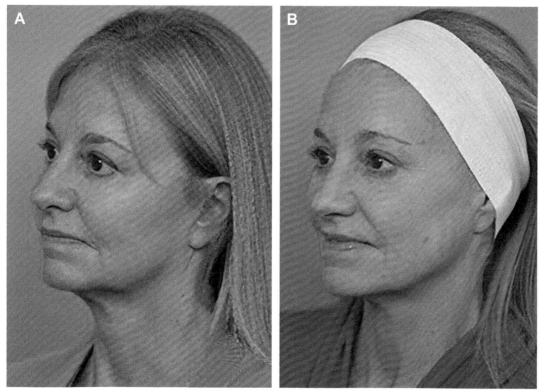

Fig. 1. Silhouette Instalift (*A*) before and (*B*) after. Improvement in oral commissure, marionette fold, and jowl.

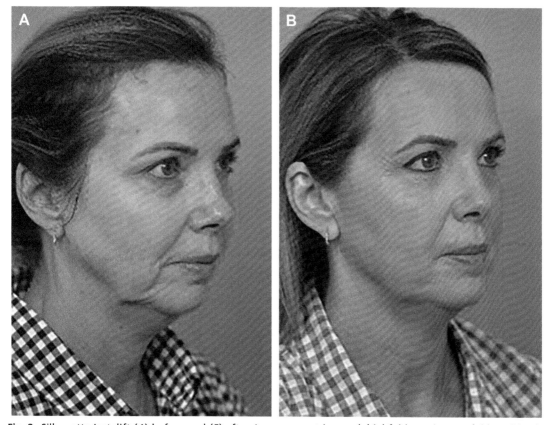

Fig. 2. Silhouette Instalift (*A*) before and (*B*) after. Improvement in nasolabial fold, marionette fold, and jowl.

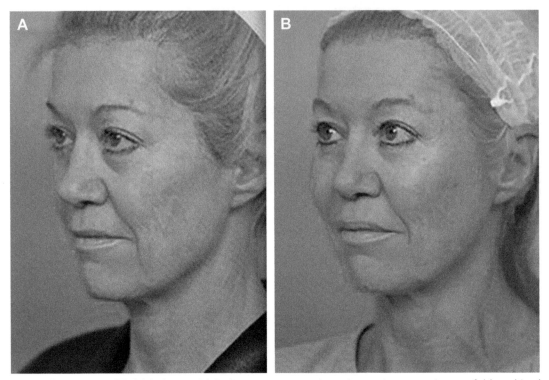

Fig. 3. Silhouette Instalift (*A*) before and (*B*) after. Improvement in oral commissure, marionette fold, and jowl. Also, note the elevated position of the cheek with reduced mid malar rhytidosis.

POLY-ʟ-LACTIC ACID

The Silhouette Instalift suture is composed of 18% PLLA. Polyglycolide or poly(glycolic acid) (PGA) was one of the first degradable polymers investigated for biomedical use.[18] It was later converted to a poly(ʟ-lactide) base for better long-term stability.[24]

Cosmetic fillers containing polylactic acid have been used to reverse signs of aging for many years.[25] This substance is unlike other dermal fillers because it does not produce immediate results. The filler is injected into the subcutaneous tissue causing the body to produce its own collagen, so results appear gradually over a period of a few months. With each treatment, there is restimulation of the recipient's own collagen. The only FDA-approved brand is Sculptra Aesthetic (Galderma Laboratories, Fort Worth, TX).[26] The company was initially Sculptra, and the product

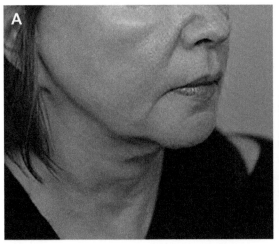
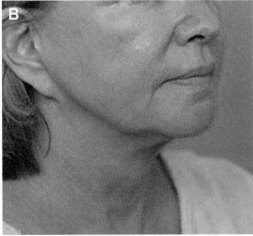

Fig. 4. Silhouette Instalift (*A*) before and (*B*) after. Improvement in jowl, marionette, and oral commissure.

Fig. 5. Silhouette Instalift sutures are equal spaced, bidirectional cones.

was approved by the FDA for use in 2004 in patients with human immunodeficiency virus for the restoration of facial features following lipoatrophy.[27] It obtained cosmetic FDA approval in 2009 for esthetic use for facial volume restoration.

PLLA is resorbed over a period of around 2 years.[18] A small number of patients, usually less than 10%, do experience the formation of subcutaneous inflammatory nodules, which are responsive to anti-inflammatory agents such as steroids.[28]

POLYLACTIDE/GLYCOLIDE

The Silhouette Instalift is composed of 82% polylactide/glycolide resorbable copolymer (PLGA). PLGA is the most investigated biodegradable polymer because of its versatility in degradation rates and its approval by the FDA for use in drug formulations and medical devices.[29] Polyglycolide and polylactide materials are widely used in medical sutures for wound closure and in orthopedic, maxillofacial, and spinal surgeries.[18]

Multiple studies report a milder soft tissue response to PLGA than with existing sutures. In the skin of rats, which is very relevant for scaffolds for skin tissue engineering, there was little to no inflammation caused by polylactide or polyglycolide materials.[30] There is no evidence of any significant cytotoxicity, systemic toxicity, genotoxicity, carcinogenicity, reproductive toxicity, or hypersensitivity with PLGA materials.[24]

DEGRADATION OF SUTURES

The Silhouette Instalift suture is a copolymer of 82% PLLA and 18% PLGA. PLLA breaks down by hydrolysis to L-lactic acid. PLGA breaks down by hydrolysis into lactic acid and glycolic acid. These products are then incorporated into normal physiologic processes and excreted.[18]

Similar to Sculptra, the sutures stimulate new type I and type III collagen as they degrade.[21] It is thought that the surrounding collagen growth encapsulates the cones and adjacent knots to help biologically fixate the suture. By doing so, the suture adds to midface volume and creates a long-lasting and contoured appearance.[15] Based on the total collagen production and fat content, along with data on European outcomes, it is believed that the results begin to peak between 3 and 6 months and may last from 18 to 36 months.[20,21] For comparison, 3 8-coned Instalift sutures contain the same amount of PLLA as 1 vial of Sculptra.[31]

SUTURE STUDIES

A study done by Sasaki and colleagues[32] in 2008 compared holding, slippage, and pull-out tension (to assess the incremental differences from the holding tension to the slippage tension) for 8 suspension sutures in the malar fat pads of fresh-frozen human cadavers. When studying the pull-out tension (a measure of the effectiveness of suture design), the tension required to remove a knotted 3 to 0 polypropylene suture with absorbable cones was significantly higher, indicating that multiple barbs provided less resistance to withdrawal than the larger cupped surfaces of the polylactide cones.[32]

After each type of suture was extracted from the soft tissue, all fixation sites on the suture were examined immediately for morphologic changes by gross magnification and by digital photography.[32] Approximately 50% of the barbs (polypropylene or polydioxanone) on each of these types of sutures demonstrated bending, curling, or stripping away from the entire length of the body of the embedded suture. To modify an intact suture into barbed suture requires micromachining cuts into the primary suture of about one-third of the diameter. Tension on the delicate barbs can cause them to bend, be stripped, and contribute to suture breakage. In contrast, all suture knot and free-standing cone sutures did not undergo any morphologic flaws after engagement, slippage, and pull-through from the soft tissues. The absorbable cones (as seen in the Silhouette Instalift suture) are free-standing units that are designed to be limited in movement by the intercalated suture knots and, therefore, do not compromise the intrinsic strength of the suture.[32]

Cappabianca[33] completed a study on collagen formation, pull-out force, and absorption rates of the Silhouette Instalift device in rat adipose tissue. The pathology conclusion was that Silhouette Instalift implants in the subcutaneous abdominal tissue of rats showed no adverse changes at 91, 182, 273, or 364 days. The implant was present and associated with formation of thin fibrous tissue (about 50–150 μm) encapsulating the entire device. There was no irritation at the implantation site. The cones showed no evidence of biodegradation at 364 days in this model, whereas the suture showed some degree of hydrolysis at 182 days that increased at 273 and 364 days and localized partial absorption.[33]

INDICATIONS AND PATIENT SELECTION

Indications for the procedure include signs of moderate midfacial tissue descent such as nasolabial folds, downturned oral commissures, and marionette folds (**Figs. 6–9**). Absorbable suture suspension should be considered for patients with mild to moderate skin laxity, men seeking nonsurgical facial rejuvenation because of facelift stigma, and those patients with contraindications for surgery such as vascular compromise or impaired wound healing. In the appropriate patient, absorbable suture suspension is a viable option compared with surgery, with an improved risk profile.[15]

CONTRAINDICATIONS

Managing expectations and proper patient selection are critical for optimal results. The sutures are not a replacement for surgery and will not achieve a facelift result. Patients with unrealistic expectations are not good candidates. The sutures should not be used in patients appearing to have very thin skin and soft tissue of the face with little to no underlying fat, in whom the implant may be visible or palpable. Patients with extensive skin laxity, thin skin, excessive skin, heavy localized rhytids, and/or malar fat sagging are not good candidates for this procedure. Patients with deep folds in the melolabial region and the

marionette region should be counseled appropriately that their response to the Silhouette Lift may be minimal.

Silhouette Instalift should not be used in patients with any known allergy or foreign body sensitivities to implant or instrument materials in particular plastic/biomaterials. The sutures should not be used in patients with active sepsis or infection, active (or history of) autoimmune disease, patients under 18 years of age, pregnant or breastfeeding women, or patients with limited ability or unwillingness to follow posttreatment recommendations.[18]

PROCEDURE

The procedure is performed in a physician's office using local anesthesia and sterile technique. The patient's face is cleansed and dried. Using a handheld mirror with the patient sitting upright, the patient and physician discuss desired movement and vectors for suture placement. Temporary markings are made using the company provided ruler of 2 exit points and 1 central entry point along the desired vectors. Three to 4 planned sutures are marked on each side of the face. To best counteract aging effects, the sutures are optimally oriented in a vector that is perpendicular to the nasolabial folds and marionette lines in a posterior/superior direction.[31] The sutures may be asymmetric to account for facial asymmetry. Local anesthetic (0.5–1 mL of 1% lidocaine with

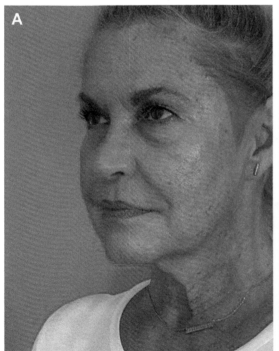
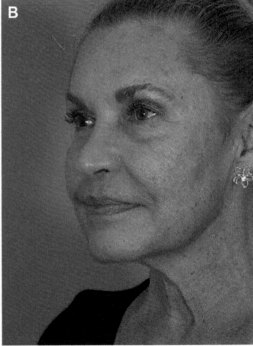

Fig. 6. Silhouette Instalift (*A*) before and (*B*) after. Improvement in marionette area and jowl.

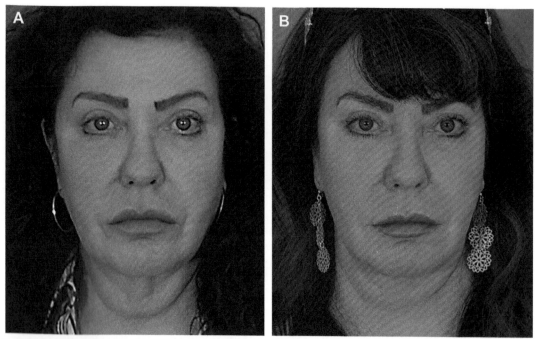

Fig. 7. Silhouette Instalift (*A*) before and (*B*) after. Improvement in nasolabial fold, marionette fold, and jowl.

epinephrine) is administered to entry and exit points. Care must be taken to mark the exit points just lateral to the downturn of the melolabial and marionette folds. Placement too far into the fold may in fact deepen the fold. The package comes with a ruler marked for 8, 12, or 16 cone uses. The exit points should be close to 4.5 cm from the central entry point.

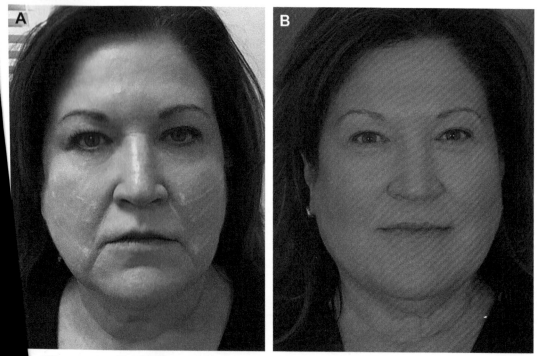

Silhouette Instalift (*A*) before and (*B*) after. Improvement in nasolabial fold, oral commissure, and mario- fold after 2 treatments, spaced 3 months apart.

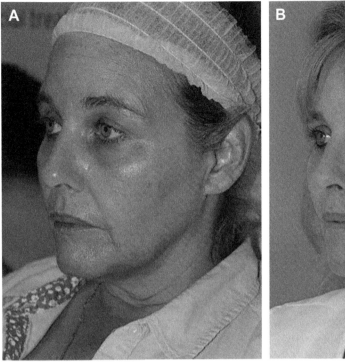
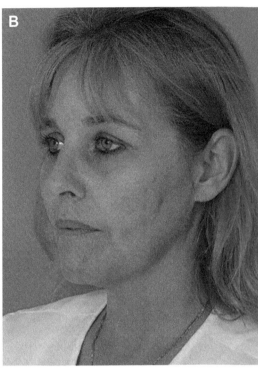

Fig. 9. Silhouette Instalift (*A*) before and (*B*) after. Improvement in oral commissure, marionette fold, and jowl.

An 18-gauge needle is used to make an insertion puncture into the subcutaneous tissue at the central entry point. Then, one of the 23-gauge suture needles is inserted vertically into this entry puncture to the depth of 5 mm until the black line on the needle disappears (**Fig. 10A**). Vertical insertion prevents dimpling at the entry point. The end of the needle is then dropped down parallel to the skin surface and advanced in the subcutaneous tissue in a linear fashion along the premarked vector. The needle then sharply punctures through the skin exit point and is pulled until the first set of cones are in place (**Fig. 10B–D**). The shape of the cone is designed to cover the knot and facilitate a smooth insertion (**Fig. 11**). This technique is repeated for the other half of the suture using the same central entry point and advancing in the opposing direction along the premarked vector (**Fig. 10E–G**). This technique is then repeated for each suture.

Once the sutures are placed under the skin, tension is applied to the suture and the soft tissue is lifted over the cones, in both directions, toward the central insertion point. When massaging the tissues over the cones, it is important to use a form of lubricant to the skin to allow for a more comfortable advancement of overlying tissues. Then the suture is pulled in the opposite direction as insertion, the knots stop the cones from slipping

to create maximum traction and tissue suspension (**Fig. 12**).[18] Excess ends of the sutures are trimmed at the skin surface to bury the end of the suture.

Although the sutures are not a "volumization" technique, by repositioning and lifting the midfacial tissues, volume is improved in the midface. Sutures may be placed in the jowls in a more vertical direction but this area is off-label, as are the neck and brows. In the neck, sutures are placed with a straight-line vector from the submental area to the postauricular area and along the jawline and lateral neck. These results have been more variable.[15] Patients should be aware that the su tures are not placed in the platysma and therefor this procedure is not a direct treatment of band but rather of ptotic subdermal tissue.

POSTPROCEDURE RECOMMENDATIONS

After the procedure, cold packs are gently ap to the face. Narcotic pain medication i required. Patients are instructed to use ace ophen. Patients should refrain from a makeup for a minimum of 24 hours. The c recommends sleeping face up in an elevat tion for 3 to 5 nights. The authors strongl mend against any therapeutic treatment the patient is face down such as mass **Fig.** face should be washed, shaved, and d *nett*

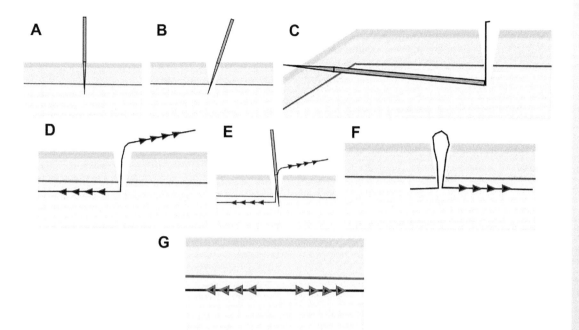

Fig. 10. Application of absorbable facial suspension sutures. (*A*) Vertical entry of the 23-gauge needle into the subdermis. (*B*) Needle is dropped horizontally to advance in the subcutaneous tissue. (*C*) Needle advances in the subcutaneous tissue until the marked exit point and then punctures through the skin. (*D*) Suture is advanced until the first set of cones are in place. (*E*) Needle is reinserted into the same central entry point and then tilted horizontally. (*F*) Suture is advanced until the second set of cones are in place. (*G*) Suture is advanced to bury cones and central cone-free zone in the subdermis.

without rubbing for 5 days. A gentle face wash is recommended for 1 to 2 days to avoid "stinging" at the open entry and exit sites. Patients should avoid high-impact sports and excessive facial/neck movements for 2 weeks, dental surgery for 3 weeks, and facial esthetic treatments for 4 weeks.[15]

WARNINGS

Care should be taken in the handling of the sutures. If the suture appears damaged before use, it should not be used. An open or damaged package should not be used. The sutures are for single use only. Re-use of this device may result in biological contamination and injury to the patient. The sutures should not be re-sterilized. Open,

unused product should be discarded according to regulatory requirements.[18]

SIDE EFFECTS

Patients should be counseled about potential side effects of the procedure. After suture placement, patients may experience minor pain, swelling, pinpoint bleeding, rippling, dimpling, and bruising.[18] These are usually temporary. Persistent bleeding at the entry or exit sites is uncommon.[22] Significant edema, asymmetry, dysesthesia, skin irregularities, or dimples are very rare (1%–2%).[22] Other potential side effects include sensory nerve injury, asymmetry, or banding.[22] Infection has not been reported in the US experience with the use of the Sinclair Pharma device.[22]

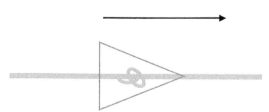

Fig. 11. Cone on insertion. The cone covers the knot during introduction.

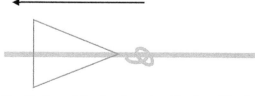

Fig. 12. Cone following insertion. The knot lifts the cone during traction.

Most complications arise from improper insertion such as not using the 18-gauge needle track for both 23 gauge needles, thereby creating a false track. Once the tip of the 23-gauge needle passes into the subcutaneous plane, it is critical to not engage the deep dermis once reoriented horizontally.[22] Sutures that are placed too deep (in the muscle) can cause pain.

A post market review was carried out for Silhouette Soft sutures on July 21, 2016. This review included all adverse events received from July 2012 to June 2016. A total of 85 adverse events were reported and an excess of 627,000 sutures were sold, resulting in an adverse event rate of 0.014% or 1 adverse event in 7378 sutures. Most events were considered minor adverse events, for example, lumps. No unacceptable risk was presented during this review.[18]

The onset of any adverse effect must be reported immediately to the company. Although the sutures are biocompatible and nontoxic, some studies have reported inflammatory reactions with the polylactide or polyglycolide implants, usually occurring 7 to 20 weeks after placement in the body.[24] The situation is closely monitored by Sinclair looking at harm levels and occurrence rates.[18]

SILHOUETTE INSTALIFT CLINICAL EXPERIENCE STUDIES

De Benito and colleagues[23] studied the Silhouette Instalift procedure in 316 patients between January 2007 and December 2009. The study demonstrated good results over a mean follow-up period of 18 months, with high patient satisfaction.[23] In 11 months, 75% of the cone material is reabsorbed suggesting full resorption of the cones after a maximum time period of 2 years.[23] All patients had stable results during the follow-up period 18 months after implantation.[23] All complications experienced by 42 patients (13.3%) were minor and temporary.[23]

Ogilvie and colleagues[15] performed a review of 100 patients treated with the Silhouette Instalift procedure. Using the Allergan Midface Volume Deficit Scale, most patients experienced 1° to 2° of improvement. Patient survey results suggest that 96% of patients reported that absorbable suture suspension is a tolerable procedure. Eighty-three percent of patients responded that the procedure was effective in improving age-related changes.[15] A total of 82% of patients were willing to recommend the procedure to friends or family.[15] This is in comparison with a study by Lycka and colleagues,[34] which showed that only 43% of patients (152 of 350 patients) described the barbed suture procedures as satisfactory.

Ogilvie and colleagues[15] found that 32% of patients who had the Silhouette Instalift procedure saw no immediate result; however, this number decreased to 17% at 3 months. In this same study, 89% of patients reported minimal to no bruising or prolonged edema that corresponded with an observed bruise rate of 6.7%.[15] There were no cases of infection requiring suture removal and no cases of asymmetry requiring revision.[15] There were no complaints of cone palpability after the first week.[15] In 2018, according to the popular cosmetic forum, RealSelf.com, the Silhouete Instalift has a satisfaction rating or "worth it" rating of 81%.[35]

In an attempt to get closer to a surgical result, physicians have combined absorbable sutures suspension with energy-based therapies (laser, ultrasound), neuromodulators, fillers, and fat transfer in the same setting. It has been reported that, as patients go through absorbable suture suspension, ptotic improvement will last around 18 months.[15] However, some physicians believe that with improved methods of placement and a stackable approach, results may last up to 36 months and beyond.[15] Whereas many physicians combine the Silhouette Instalift with other therapies and injectables products, it is important to note that clinical research and recommendations have not been established for combined therapies. Additional sutures may be placed after the initial procedure. With recent research on the delayed improvement from collagen stimulation, results are now reassessed at least 3–6 months after the procedure before proceeding with additional sutures.

In 2017, an expert consensus on absorbable advanced suspension technology for facial tissue repositioning and volume enhancement was published by Nestor and colleagues.[22] Their study concluded that, when performed properly, absorbable facial suspension is associated with minor and infrequent complications and is a beneficial clinical alternative to traditional facial rejuvenation techniques. They reported that results generally peak after 5 to 6 months and are maintained for 1.5 to 2 years.[36] A study on vector planning and optimal results was published in 2018 by Lorenc and colleagues.[31] Together, the authors have performed over 500 procedures since FDA approval.[31] They report that there have been no adverse effects and that noticeable bruising has occurred in less than 5% of patients.[31]

PRACTICE MANAGEMENT

An extensive knowledge of facial anatomy is important for this procedure. To perform the

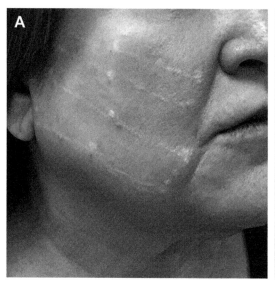 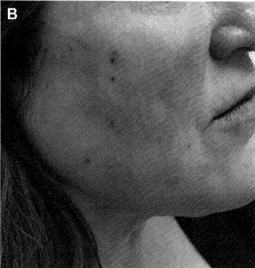

Fig. 13. (*A*) Heavy nasolabial fold and marionette fold with markings for 4 sutures. (*B*) Immediately after insertion of 4 sutures with improvement of the nasolabial fold and marionette fold.

Silhouette Instalift, a provider must attend a 1-day training session hosted by the company in designated cities across the country. At present this training is only offered to physicians.

It is important to educate everyone in the office about the new procedure but especially if the office has injectors and estheticians who provide alternative revenue streams/service lines. Most likely, they will already know patients who would be excellent candidates—loyal patients with some facial deflation and gravity changes who get fillers on a regular basis but are not seeing as much "lifting" as they would like from these treatments. As facial plastic surgeons, it is imperative that patients are counseled on all the possible treatments for the aging lower face. It is also important to clearly state the inherent differences in treatments with the individual pitfalls for each.

The sutures are relatively expensive. Each suture costs $150 and comes in a sterile pack of 2 sutures. For 4 sutures on each side of the face, the product cost is $1200. The minimum purchase is a box of 5 packs (10 sutures) at $1500.

To advertise the procedure, practices have reached out to local TV stations about the "latest and greatest" in minimally invasive techniques, local magazines/print, and used social media/digital media. Offices have filmed live demonstration videos for YouTube and performed live demonstration events. The company provides "swag" including posters for the waiting room/treatment rooms as well as brochures. The company also offers digital marketing materials including high-resolution pictures of the sutures, logos, and short videos. Introducing the Silhouette Instalift can also be a way for practices to become more involved with local charities and/or nonprofit organizations by donating a portion of proceeds from the procedure to these groups.

When discussing any version of a thread or suture procedure to patients, it is our experience that most of them are wary of the negative press from thread lifts of the past. It is important to discuss why the Silhouette Instalift procedure is different from the predecessors. The Silhouette Instalift offers a nonsurgical approach to reposition descended midfacial tissues with minimal downtime and immediate results (**Fig. 13**). The most important part of education is in showing the benefit of nonpermanence. The "threads" will absorb and become replaced with collagen production holding the tissues in place for up to 24 months. Patients can be back to work the next day. The sutures use cones and knots rather than barbs. Not only are the cones and sutures fully resorbable, but provide added benefit through the documented collagen-stimulating abilities of PLLA and PLGA. This bio-stimulatory property allows the sutures to also address age-related volume loss.[31] Importantly, the procedure has been shown in multiple studies to have a very high safety profile.

SUMMARY

Absorbable suture suspension is one of the newest minimally invasive treatment trends for lifting and repositioning ptotic facial tissue. The

Silhouette Instalift is a convenient in-office procedure that provides a unique and advanced clinical treatment for a natural looking midfacial lift. The PLLA and PLGA materials have several decades of clinical success in many areas including esthetics with a safe clinical profile. Research has shown that most patients characterized the Silhouette Instalift as tolerable, immediately effective, and most were consistently pleased by the natural enhancements. The procedure has an improved safety and efficacy profile over the predecessor, barbed suture thread lifting, coupled with a reduced risk of complications and recovery time compared with a rhytidectomy. Absorbable suture suspension should be considered a workhorse in nonsurgical aesthetic treatments.

REFERENCES

1. Cosmetic surgery national data bank statistics. Aesthet Surg J 2017;37(suppl 2):1–29.
2. Sulamanidze MA, Shiffman MA, Paikidze TG, et al. Facial lifting with APTOS threads. Int J Cosmet Surg Aesthet Dermatol 2001;3:275–81.
3. Sulamanidze MA, Fournier PF, Paikidze TG, et al. Removal of facial soft tissue ptosis with special threads. Dermatol Surg 2002;28:367–71.
4. Kaminer MS, Mandy S. ContourLift™: a new method of minimally invasive facial rejuvenation. J Cosmet Dermatol 2007;20:29–35.
5. Sulamanidze MA, Paikidze TG, Sulamanidze GM, et al. Facial lifting with "APTOS" threads: featherlift. Otolaryngol Clin North Am 2005;38(5):1109–17.
6. Lee S, Isse N. Barbed polypropylene sutures for midface elevation: early results. Arch Facial Plast Surg 2005;7(1):55–61.
7. Wu WT. Barbed sutures in facial rejuvenation. Aesthet Surg J 2004;24(6):582–7.
8. DeLorenzi C. Barbed sutures: rationale and technique. Aesthet Surg J 2006;26:223–9.
9. Paul MD. Using barbed sutures in open/subperiosteal midface lifting. Aesthet Surg J 2006;26(6): 725–32.
10. Rachel JD, Lack EB, Larson B. Incidence of complications and early recurrence in 29 patients after facial rejuvenation with barbed suture lifting. Dermatol Surg 2010;36(3):348–54.
11. Villa MT, White LE, Alam M, et al. Barbed sutures: a review of the literature. Plast Reconstr Surg 2008; 121(3):102e–8e.
12. Paul MD. Complications of barbed sutures. Aesthetic Plast Surg 2008;32(1):149.
13. Garvey PB, Ricciardelli EJ, Gampper T. Outcomes in threadlift for facial rejuvenation. Ann Plast Surg 2009;62(5):482–5.
14. Samalonis LB. Midface elevation technique: early results using barbed polypropylene sutures for midface elevation are promising. Cosmetic Surgery Times 2005;8:33.
15. Ogilvie MP, Few JW, Tomur SS, et al. Rejuvenating the face: an analysis of 100 absorbable suture suspension patients. Aesthet Surg J 2018;38(6):654–63.
16. Abraham RF, DeFatta RJ, Williams EF. Thread-lift for facial rejuvenations – assessment of long term results. Arch Facial Plast Surg 2009;11:178–83.
17. Available at: http://www.silhouette-soft.com/how-it-works. Accessed January 15, 2017.
18. Trumbic B. Silhouette Soft® safety: safety data report. Silhouette Instalift Inc.: Irvine, CA; 2016.
19. Available at: https://www.accessdata.fda.gov/scripts/cdrh/cfdocs/cfpmn/pmn.cfm?ID=K142061. Accessed June 6, 2018.
20. Instruction Packet-Instalift. Available at: http://www.instalift.com. Accessed September 28, 2017.
21. Goldberg D, Guana A, Volk A, et al. Single-arm study for the characterization of human tissue response to injectable poly-L-lactic acid. Dermatol Surg 2013;39(6):915–22.
22. Nestor MS, Ablong G, Andriessen A, et al. Expert consensus on absorbable advanced suspension technology for facial tissue repositioning and volume enhancement. J Drugs Dermatol 2017;16(7):661–6.
23. De Benito J, Pizzamiglio R, Theodorou D, et al. Facial rejuvenation and improvement of malar projection using sutures with absorbable cones: surgical technique and case series. Aesthetic Plast Surg 2011;35(2):248–53.
24. Williams D. The biocompatibility, biological safety and clinical applications of PURASORB® resorbable polymers. An independent report compiled for Purac Biomaterials. 2010. Available at: http://geomedicspharma.com/wp-content/uploads/2017/07/14.The-Biocompatibility-Biological-Safety-and-Clinical-Applications-of-sutures.pdf. Accessed August 15, 2018.
25. Palm MD, Woodhall KE, Butterwick KJ, et al. Cosmetic use of poly-L-lactic acid: a retrospective study of 130 patients. Dermatol Surg 2010;36(2): 161–70.
26. American Society of Plastic Surgeons. Dermal fillers: polylactic acid. Minimally invasive procedure. 2016. Available at: http://www.plasticsurgery.org/cosmetic-procedures/dermal-fillers-polylactic-acid.html#content. Accessed August 15, 2018.
27. Burgess CM, Quiroga RM. Assessment of the safety and efficacy of poly-L-lactic acid for the treatment of HIV-associated facial lipoatrophy. J Am Acad Dermatol 2005;52(2):233–9.
28. Ulery BD, Nair LS, Laurencin CT. Biomedical applications of biodegradable polymers. J Polym Sci B Polym Phys 2011;49(12):832–64.
29. Taluja A, Youn YS, Bae YH. Novel approaches in microparticulate PLGA delivery systems encapsulating proteins. J Mater Chem 2007;17(38):4002–14.

30. Cooper ML, Hansbrough JF, Spielvogel RL, et al. In vivo optimization of a living dermal substitute employing cultured human fibroblasts on a biodegradable polyglycolic acid or polyglactin mesh. Biomaterials 1991;12(2):243–8.

31. Lorenc ZP, Goldberg D, Nestor M. Straight-line vector planning for optimal results with Silhouette InstaLift in minimally invasive tissue repositioning for facial rejuvenation. J Drugs Dermatol 2018; 17(7):786–93.

32. Sasaki GH, Komorowska-Timek ED, Bennett BC, et al. An objective comparison of holding, slippage, and pull-out tensions for eight suspension sutures in the malar fat pads of fresh-frozen human cadavers. Aesthet Surg J 2008;28(4):387–96.

33. Cappabianca L. Silhouette Instalift device absorption rate and pull-out evaluation in rat adipose tissue – GLP study. DaVinci Biomedical Research Products; 2014.

34. Lycka B, Bazan C, Poletti E, et al. The emerging technique of the antiptosis subdermal suspension thread. Dermatol Surg 2004;30(1):41–4 [discussion: 44].

35. Available at: https://www.realself.com/silhouette-instalift. Accessed June 1, 2018.

36. Nicolau PJ. Use of suspending threads in facial rejuvenation. Prime 2014;September:50–6.

Advanced Techniques in Nonsurgical Rhinoplasty

Umang Mehta, MD[a],*, Zachary Fridirici, MD[b]

KEYWORDS

- Rhinoplasty • Nose • Filler • Nonsurgical rhinoplasty • Injection rhinoplasty • Hyaluronic acid fillers
- Advanced techniques • Tip rotation

KEY POINTS

- Nonsurgical rhinoplasty represents a safe and efficacious treatment when filler is placed in the nose carefully and judiciously.
- The injector must have an intimate knowledge of the nasal vascular anatomy and understand what to do in situations of vascular compromise.
- Hyaluronic acid filler in the nose can be used for dorsal augmentation as well as camouflaging of the nasal hump.
- Advanced techniques include increasing tip rotation and projection, straightening the nose, lowering alar rims, and perhaps improving nasal valve function.

 Video content accompanies this article at http://www.facialplastic.theclinics.com.

INTRODUCTION

With the increasing demand for nonsurgical alternatives and the continued popularity of rhinoplasty (the third most common cosmetic surgical procedure), patient requests for nonsurgical rhinoplasty continue to increase.[1] It is of paramount importance that facial plastic surgeons are adept and comfortable with filler placement in the nose for a multitude of reasons.

First, facial plastic surgeons who perform surgical rhinoplasty have the most profound knowledge of nasal anatomy. This knowledge is critical for the safety and efficacy of filler placement. The optimal approach to nonsurgical rhinoplasty necessitates thinking in terms of grafts used during rhinoplasty, rather than just contour changes.

Second, this treatment is being performed by nonsurgeon physicians and midlevel providers.

By offering this treatment, facial plastic surgeons are providing patients with a safer alternative to injectors who may be less experienced.

Third, nonsurgical rhinoplasty helps to drive a successful surgical rhinoplasty practice. Many patients who present for nasal fillers may not be optimal candidates. Computer imaging can help patients understand the benefits and limitations of nonsurgical versus surgical rhinoplasty. Others may be considering surgery in the future, in which case nonsurgical rhinoplasty can help build confidence in the surgeon and provide an opportunity to "test drive" their new nose for several months or years.

The fourth consideration is duration. In the authors' experience, nasal filler can last 1 to 2 years or more with a single session. This time duration makes it cost-effective for patients, because 12 to 15 sessions of nonsurgical rhinoplasty over

Disclosure Statement: There are no financial conflicts or interests to disclose.
[a] Mehta Plastic Surgery, 3351 El Camino Real, Suite 205, Atherton, CA 94027, USA; [b] Department of Otolaryngology, Head and Neck Surgery, University of California San Francisco, 2320 Sutter, Suite 102, San Francisco, CA 94115, USA
* Corresponding author.
E-mail address: drmehta@mehtaplastics.com

Facial Plast Surg Clin N Am 27 (2019) 355–365
https://doi.org/10.1016/j.fsc.2019.04.008

several years may be performed before reaching the cost of a surgical rhinoplasty. Limited downtime and risk associated with nasal fillers may make them an attractive long-term solution. These benefits are particularly true of patients with smaller noses, lower dorsums, and shorter septums, for whom primary nasal surgery may necessitate ear or rib cartilage harvest.

Fifth, rhinoplasty surgeons may find placement of filler following rhinoplasty to be invaluable. The ability to smooth minor nasal contour indentations or rotate/project/straighten the tip can help to reduce the likelihood of revision rhinoplasty and its associated expenses, risks, and downtime.

Overall, nonsurgical rhinoplasty offers a quick, safe, and effective treatment, if the proper filler is placed judiciously. This article provides an overview of the relevant nasal vascular anatomy, discusses safety considerations in nonsurgical rhinoplasty, explores complications related to nasal filler placement, and reviews both basic and advanced techniques.

Nasal Vascular Anatomy

An intimate knowledge of nasal anatomy is paramount to the safe practice of nonsurgical rhinoplasty. The nasal framework is draped by a soft tissue envelope comprising 5 layers that overlie the perichondrium or periosteum base. From superficial to deep, these layers are the epidermis, dermis, superficial fatty layer, fibromuscular layer (continuation of the superficial musculoaponeurotic system [SMAS]), and deep fatty layer (**Fig. 1**).[2]

The vascular network of the nose originates from both the external and the internal carotid arteries via the facial artery and ophthalmic artery, respectively.[3] The facial artery and its course along the nasolabial fold are categorized as 1 of 3 types, as described by Saban and colleagues.[3] In their study using cadavers and ultrasound imaging, they found that in 80% of the cases the artery coursed medial to the nasolabial fold (type I). In 15% of the cases, the artery coursed into the cheek, lateral to the nasolabial fold (type II). In 5% of cases, they found the facial artery terminated in the parasymphyseal region, with the contralateral facial artery providing vascular supply to both sides of the nose (type III). There are 4 constant arteries: the subnasal artery, angular artery, dorsal nasal artery, and lateral nasal artery, as depicted in **Fig. 2**.

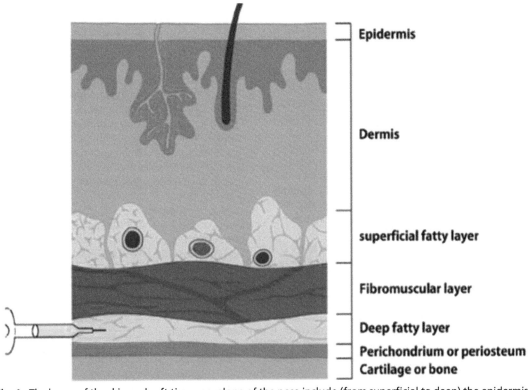

Fig. 1. The layers of the skin and soft tissue envelope of the nose include (from superficial to deep) the epidermis, dermis, superficial fatty layer, fibromuscular layer, and deep fatty layer. Underneath the skin/soft tissue envelope lie the perichondrium or periosteum and the cartilage or bone.

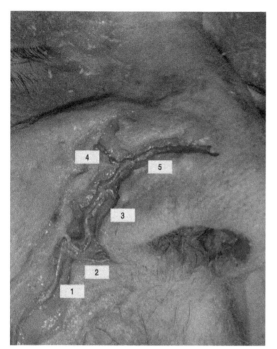

Fig. 2. Nasal branches of the facial artery. Dissection of the main branches of the facial artery, showing the initial step in the dissection of the facial artery and its main branches. The facial artery (1) is visible lateral to the oral commissure; it then forms the subnasal artery (2), marginal alar artery (3), angular artery (4), and lateral nasal artery (5). (*From* Saban Y, Andretto Amodeo C, Bouaziz D, et al. Nasal Arterial Vasculature: medical and surgical applications. Arch Facial Plast Surg 2012;14(6): 429-36; with permission.)

The subnasal artery branches at the alar-facial recess and courses medially to the lower columella, where it extends superiorly to the nasal tip as the columellar artery (anastomosis with philtral artery from the superior labial artery). The marginal artery is a terminal branch of the facial artery (83%) or lateral nasal artery coursing along the caudal border of the lower lateral cartilage (LLC). The marginal artery shares multiple anastomotic arcades with the lateral nasal artery over the lateral crus of the LLC. The lateral nasal artery, as described by Toriumi and colleagues,[4] courses along the cephalic border of the LLC and anastomoses with the columellar arteries at the nasal tip. The angular artery runs vertically toward the medial canthus, where it anastomoses with the ophthalmic arterial system. The internal carotid system gives rise to the ophthalmic artery, and therefore, the dorsal nasal artery anastomotic arcade. The dorsal nasal artery runs vertically along the dorsum of the nose, whereas the radix artery is oriented horizontally, with branches anastomosing to the contralateral system.

Saban and colleagues[3] simplify the arterial supply to the nose into a polygonal system based on 4 transfacial arcades. The intercarotid anastomosis of the angular and dorsal arteries provides the vertical systems with the radix, lateral nasal, marginal, and subnasal artery providing the horizontal or transfacial anastomoses (**Fig. 3**).

SAFETY

Besides knowledge of nasal vascular anatomy, safe nonsurgical rhinoplasty necessitates selection of the optimal filler as well as placement with the proper technique, depth, and locations.

A multitude of fillers have been placed in the nose.[5] These fillers include hyaluronic acid (HA) fillers, calcium hydroxyapatite, liquid silicone, and polymethyl methacrylate, among others. When selecting a filler, one must consider reversibility,

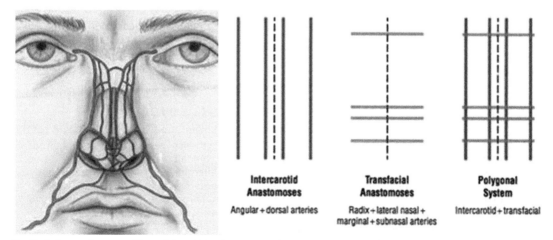

Fig. 3. Polygonal system. (*From* Saban Y, Andretto Amodeo C, Bouaziz D, et al. Nasal Arterial Vasculature: medical and surgical applications. Arch Facial Plast Surg 2012;14(6): 429-36; with permission.)

duration, and stiffness. Reversibility is paramount in terms of safety. When arterial insufficiency or venous congestion is suspected, reversal of the filler may help to alleviate these issues or minimize their sequelae. For this reason, HA fillers are the optimal choices for nonsurgical rhinoplasty.

HA fillers bring an additional benefit over calcium hydroxyapatite. If surgery is performed after a patient has had prior nonsurgical rhinoplasty, HA fillers are reversible if they have not yet resorbed. They are also easily removed during surgery, if needed. In addition, the tissue planes remain clean and easily separated during surgery. Calcium hydroxyapatite tends to create additional fibrosis, which can add complexity to the lifting of the skin and soft tissue envelope.

The safest injection depth is in the rhinoplasty plane of dissection, just superficial to the perichondrium and periosteum. The vascular plexus of the nose should obviously be avoided. Depth of injection can be determined by placing the needle or cannula down on the level of the bone and cartilage.

Nasal filler should be injected very slowly, while carefully watching for skin color changes. Aspiration before injection is critical as well. A flash of blood in the syringe indicates intravascular introduction of the needle tip. Filler must not be pushed forward immediately following this flash. One should remove the needle, apply pressure, and then reintroduce it from a different entry point and at a different depth.

"Danger zones" of the nose include the area just lateral to the alar facial junction, nasal tip, alar rims, alar creases, and the area superior to the nose, in the glabella. Injection in these areas necessitates even greater caution, and the decision of whether or not to inject should be weighed more carefully.

CANNULA USE

When possible, use of blunt cannulas may reduce the risk of intravascular injection, although there have been reports of blindness and skin necrosis despite cannula use. In the senior author's practice, cannulas are useful in areas such as the tear troughs, cheeks, and nasal dorsum, where the number of needle introduction points can be minimized. Cannulas should result in reduced bruising, both from atraumatic passage through tissue and from fewer skin penetrations.

For the nose, cannula use is most useful for long, straight vectors of placement, such as a continuous dorsum without a significant hump. In the senior author's practice, the 27-gauge cannula is used for most indications. The cannula port should be directed away from the skin envelope.

Cannula use should not obviate other safety considerations, such as depth, location, and aspiration.

COMPLICATIONS

Nonsurgical rhinoplasty is a generally safe procedure, with most complications avoided through patient selection, product selection, and practicing the techniques mentioned above. Complication rates are low, but need to be thoroughly discussed with patients before injection (**Table 1**).

The most severe, major complication of nonsurgical rhinoplasty is vascular compromise, which has the potential for dermal necrosis and blindness. The mechanism is categorized as extravascular, intravascular, or combined. Extravascular compromise is due to filler producing a mass effect and vascular compression (specifically venous). Intravascular compromise is secondary to injection of filler into the vessel lumen with subsequent direct obstruction, embolism, or endothelial damage.[6] During injection, the surgeon must be vigilant to watch for dermal blanching with or without complaints of severe, spreading pain. Local tissue ischemia progresses to geographic (vascular territory) edema, erythema, and necrosis. Furthermore, intra-arterial injection (especially under high pressure) carries the risk of retrograde arterial embolism to the ophthalmic and retinal artery with the potential of ocular issues and blindness.

Early recognition and intervention are critical in the setting of vascular compromise. If any signs are noted, injections should be ceased and filler dissolved.[7] All clinics should have an Emergency Kit (**Box 1**) ready, to permit rapid intervention with massage, warm compresses, 2% nitroglycerin paste, hyaluronidase injection, and aspirin administration. High-dose hyaluronidase injection (200–300 U) should be performed to the entire

Table 1 Immediate and delayed complications following filler injection	
Immediate (<24 h)/Early (24 h to 4 wk)	**Delayed (>4 wk)**
Edema, erythema, itching, Tyndall effect, allergic reaction, inflammatory nodules, herpes outbreak, vascular compromise	Granulomatous inflammation, foreign body reaction, migration of the filler, scarring, asymmetry, discoloration

area, with repeat injection hourly until clinical resolution is achieved or doses nearing 1500 U have been reached.[8] Injections should then be performed daily until signs or symptoms are reversed. Adjunct procedures, such as oxygen administration or hyperbaric oxygen treatments, should be strongly considered. Some resources advocate for the injection of 10 μg of prostaglandin E1 daily for 5 days.[9] After the initial time period, local wound care and antibiotic therapy may be indicated. Critical to any major, procedural complication is a solid rapport and open communication with the patient.

Vision loss or changes indicate retrograde embolism affecting the retinal artery. In the event of central retinal artery occlusion, irreversible changes and blindness occur within 60 to 90 minutes.[10] All of the above measures should be performed with the addition of ocular massage (firm pressure to a closed eye for 5 seconds with a quick release), 1 drop of topical timolol 0.5%, sublingual nitroglycerin 0.6 mg, rebreathing into a paper bag, and rapid referral to an ophthalmology center, for possible retrobulbar injection of hyaluronidase, anterior chamber paracentesis, steroids, and mannitol.[11]

Early hyaluronidase administration (<4 hours) is critical. Delayed (>24 hours) injection efficacy is still a point of controversy anecdotally and in animal model studies[12] (see **Box 1**).

GENERAL PRINCIPLES OF NONSURGICAL RHINOPLASTY

In the nose, fillers with a higher G′ tend to be more effective than those with a lower G′. G′ is known as the elastic modulus, and it is a representation of the ability of a filler to resist deformation. Stiffer fillers, such as a high G′, large-particle HA gel, more closely mimic natural bone and cartilage, yielding results that are more defined, precise, and sharp. Softer, more pliable fillers can provide

width to the placement areas without as much height or definition (**Fig. 3**).

BASIC TECHNIQUES
Dorsal Augmentation

When performing nonsurgical rhinoplasty, one should think in terms of cartilage grafts, rather than simply contour. On the dorsum, filler placement is an alternative to surgical diced cartilage placement. Patients with a low dorsum, most typically those of Asian or African descent, often desire a taller, narrower-appearing dorsum. These patients often have a shorter quadrangular cartilage, and ear or rib cartilage may be needed, even in primary rhinoplasty. Even with meticulous surgical technique, dorsal diced cartilage grafts may result in minor contour irregularities as the skin and soft tissue envelope shrinks back down. The smoothness and ease of dorsal filler placement may make this an attractive alternative.

In patients with a lower dorsum, it is important to consider the natural nasal starting point, typically at the midpupillary line. Computer simulation can be helpful to determine whether the patient is seeking this lower starting point or one which sits at the level of the superior lid crease.

To fill the dorsum, one may use a cannula, introduced in the supratip. The bevel is placed downward toward the perichondrium or periosteum. If the cannula is in the proper plane, it should glide easily. There have been cases of blindness reported in the literature with injections in and around the radix/glabella.[11] For this reason, it is recommended to tent the skin/soft tissue envelope up while keeping one's fingers along the nasal sidewalls. This technique also keeps the product in the midline. The cannula tip should be kept below the level of the nasion. The product can be massaged upwards easily after injection, if desired.

In most patients, 0.4 to 0.6 mL of filler is enough to provide enough dorsal height, depending on the native height and the desired effect. A dorsal hump can be created with filler. Increased tip projection may be advisable when augmenting the dorsum, to avoid a hooked-appearing profile (**Fig. 4**).

CAMOUFLAGING A HUMP

Reduction of the nasal hump is the most common request in surgical rhinoplasty. It follows that this is a common request in nonsurgical rhinoplasty as well. Many patients who present for this maneuver may actually be better surgical candidates, especially in the case of a large hump or a shallower radix. Computer imaging can be a helpful way to

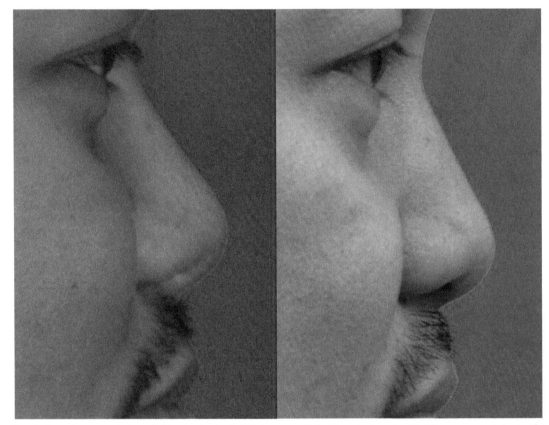

Fig. 4. Dorsal augmentation: 0.55 mL of a high G0, large-particle HA gel placed with 27-gauge cannula on the dorsum and 0.15 mL placed at tip.

illustrate this to patients, because a very tall radix may be undesirable.

Placement of filler above and below the dorsal hump is a straightforward maneuver. If the hump is small, this can be done with a cannula in the supratip. For larger humps, placement at 2 points may be indicated, cephalad and caudal. A 29-gauge needle is most commonly used in the senior author's practice for this placement. Placement of the filler at the proper depth and aspiration, in particular at the radix, is very important. Depending on hump size relative to the radix, 0.2 to 0.3 mL of filler cephalic and 0.1 to 0.2 mL distal to the hump are generally sufficient.

Similar to dorsal augmentation, the natural nasal starting point must be assessed. Distally, some patients desire a supratip break, whereas others prefer a straight dorsum (**Fig. 5**).

ADVANCED TECHNIQUES

More experienced injectors may elect to perform advanced nasal filler maneuvers. These maneuvers require deeper consideration of the safety factors previously discussed, including injection depth and vascular anatomy. That said, these techniques can be safely and effectively performed, providing patients with predictable results that can approximate, to some extent, what can be achieved with nasal surgery.

Tip Rotation

Rotation of a droopy nasal tip is a common request of patients who present to a facial plastic surgery office. A ptotic tip can cause an aged appearance, because the nasal tip tends to counterrotate with time. In addition, feminine noses may appear more masculine if the tip is ptotic. The ideal tip angle for feminine noses is 95° to 105°, whereas this same angle should be 90° to 95° for male noses.

The Tripod Theory is a well-established principle in rhinoplasty.[13] Each lateral crus represents 1 leg of the tripod, whereas the paired medial crura represent the third. Rotation of the tip can be accomplished by shortening the lateral crura with an overlay procedure, lengthening the medial crura, or setting the entire tripod on a more prominent base. Surgically, the senior author uses a

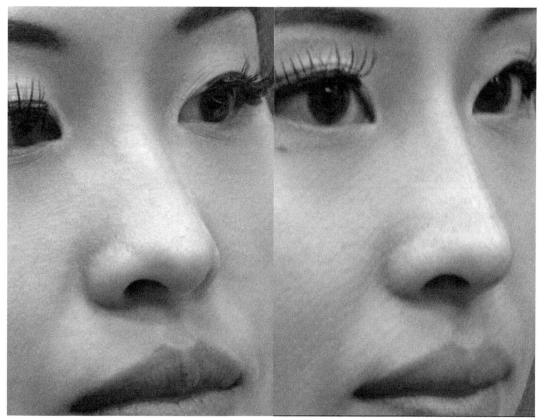

Fig. 5. Camouflaging a hump: 0.25 mL of a high G0, large-particle HA gel placed proximal to the hump and 0.25 mL placed distal in lower dorsum. Also, 0.2 mL is placed at the tip to increase projection and 0.25 mL placed at the base of the columella for rotation.

caudal septal extension graft and septocolumellar suture for this latter effect, offering predictable and durable tip rotation and projection.

Nonsurgically, the medial crural leg of the trip can be effectively lengthened with placement of filler under the base of the medial crura, in the area of the footplates. Typically 0.15 to 0.2 mL is required for this maneuver. The filler advances the medial crural footplates anteriorly as well, reducing the degree of overlap of these footplates with the septum. This placement lengthens the base of the columella slightly, which can be advantageous in patients with a mildly retracted base.

The filler is introduced from an anterior approach directly at the base of the columella. The filler is placed deep, near the posterior septal angle, to avoid injection near or into the columellar arteries, which are superficial. Aspiration is also important. The injector should place his or her fingers on each side of the medial crural footplates, to avoid splaying them. The amount of filler should generally not exceed 0.2 mL, because a large bolus may compromise the external valves and widen the columellar base.

Tip Projection

Tip projection is a complex and critical concept in both surgical and nonsurgical rhinoplasty. Goode's ratio has been used to describe ideal tip projection relative to the distance from the nasion to the subnasale.[14] The ratio of tip projection to this nasion/columellar base distance should be 0.55 to 0.6, approximating a perfect 3-4-5 right triangle.

Increasing tip projection in medium- or thicker-skinned patients can offer a significant improvement in tip definition. A rounder tip can be made more triangular. A firmer, prominent tip structure can be thought of as pushing into a thicker skin envelope. Surgically, this is achieved with caudal septal extension grafts, septocolumellar sutures, shield grafts, and tip grafts.

Filler placement at the tip is achieved by placing 0.1 to 0.15 mL of filler in front of the tip-defining points, precisely in the midline. The optimal approach is from an entry point in the infratip, using a 29-gauge needle. The skin and soft tissue envelope can be tented up to reduce risk of intravascular injection. Aspiration is important, of course. The filler should be placed very slowly, immediately upon the perichondrium of the tip cartilages. The filler can then be shaped with the fingers. If desired, the infratip can be slightly lengthened using this technique as well, if the filler is in the form of a shield graft. A small amount of additional filler in the supratip may be advisable, if the increased projection accentuates the supratip break (**Fig. 6**) (Video 1).

Straightening the Nose

Because facial symmetry has long been perceived as aesthetically desirable, a crooked nose can be problematic. Deviation of the nose can occur at the upper dorsum, lower dorsum, and tip, and often some combination of all 3. Surgically, straightening the upper dorsum of the nose often requires medial and lateral osteotomies, with possible spreader graft placement to support the previously infractured nasal bone and narrowed upper lateral cartilage. A unilateral spreader graft or bilateral grafts of different width are used to straighten the middle vault, and the mid and lower dorsum. Clocking sutures can also be helpful.

Finally, at the tip, it is important to properly assess the cause of the tip deviation. Most commonly, this occurs due to deviation of the caudal septum, in which case a caudal septal repositioning or reconstruction may be required. A caudal septal extension graft is also often used in the senior author's practice, to create a midline point to which the tip can be attached.

Differential heights of the premaxilla on each side can also contribute to tip deviation. During the consultation, the surgeon should palpate the premaxilla bilaterally to determine if there is a unilateral deficiency. Often the ala appears higher and smaller on the affected side, in what has been called the "hidden ala syndrome." Augmentation of the affected side with cartilage or filler can create more symmetry on front and base views, while straightening the nasal tip. Surgically, this is done with a few small fragments of cartilage placed under the alar base through an intranasal incision and is commonly known as a premaxillary or subnasal graft.

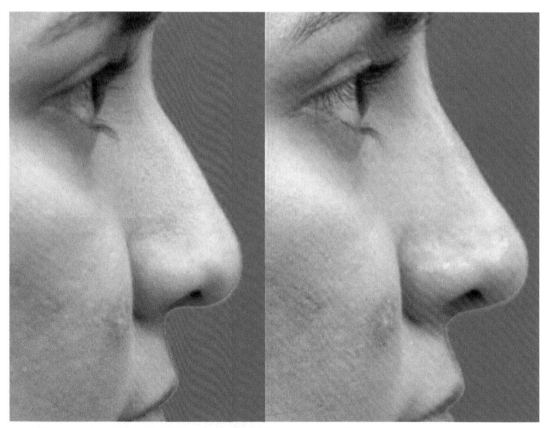

Fig. 6. Tip rotation and projection: 0.15 mL of a high G, large-particle HA gel placed at the base of the columella to increase tip rotation, and 0.2 mL placed at the tip, for projection. Also, 0.35 mL was placed proximal to the hump and 0.1 mL distal to the hump in the lower dorsum.

Straightening the nose with filler is quite straightforward. The filler can be placed on the concave side of the nasal bones or middle vault. The filler is effectively being used to create a spreader graft. Because this may widen the dorsum, proper patient selection (those with a thinner dorsum), frank counseling, and computer imaging can help.

Correction of a premaxillary deficiency is another useful application of nonsurgical rhinoplasty. The product is placed is deep on the maxilla. The needle should enter through a medial location, at the junction of the ala and the upper lip, rather than laterally, where the ala meets the cheek. The marginal and lateral nasal arteries are at risk with a lateral introduction. Aspiration of the 29-gauge needle when upon the periosteum of the maxilla is advisable before injection. Approximately 0.2 to 0.3 mL of filler is needed, depending on the degree of premaxillary deficiency. This placement is generally done unilaterally to straighten the tip, although bilateral placement could be done in patients with an underdeveloped, retrusive maxilla (**Fig. 7**).

Lowering Alar Rims

Alar retraction can be congenital, traumatic, or iatrogenic, with the latter of these being the most common. Overresection or malpositioning of the LLCs can cause the alar rim to retract, increasing columellar show. A hanging columella may also increase columellar show, so it is important to assess whether this is also a contributing factor.

Surgically, alar rims can be lowered by placing rim grafts, strut grafts, or composite grafts or with a repositioning the lateral crus. Strengthening this area can also reduce pinching of the tip and improve external valve patency.

Filler can also be placed along the alar rim, achieving some of the same effects as a rim graft. The filler is introduced laterally with a 29-gauge needle, slowly and with frequent aspiration. Particular care should be taken in patients who have undergone prior rhinoplasty, because the normal marginal arterial flow may already be compromised. When in the proper plane, the needle moves forward relatively effortlessly. Overall, this is a somewhat risky area of placement, so it should only be performed by experienced

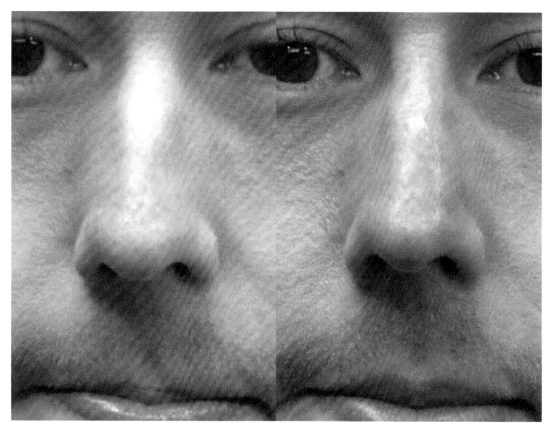

Fig. 7. Straightening the nose: 0.35 mL of a high G0, large-particle HA gel was placed in the right premaxillary area, 0.5 mL in the left middle vault, and 0.5 mL placed proximal to the hump. Filler was placed over 2 sessions, spaced one week apart.

injectors with proper precautions. Composite graft placement (under local anesthesia +/- oral sedation) is an alternative to filler for lowering alar rims (**Fig. 8**).

FUNCTIONAL APPLICATIONS

Narrow internal or external valves, either at rest or during inspiration, can cause nasal obstruction. Surgically, a variety of approaches have been used to improve the valves, including spreader grafts, autospreader grafts, butterfly grafts, alar batten grafts, strut grafts, alar spanning sutures, composite grafts, bone-anchored suture fixation, and rim grafts.

An implant consisting of poly-L-lactic acid (Latera) has been used for nasal valve collapse.[15] Although studies show effectiveness, there could be some potential benefits or disadvantages of HA fillers versus Latera. The first benefit is patient comfort, because Latera deployment requires injection of local anesthetic followed by introduction and advancement of a large cannula. Latera carries a small risk of implant extrusion or visibility through the skin. Cost must also be considered, because the price of a syringe of filler is perhaps one-third that of the implant. The final factor is longevity. It is unclear if the stiffness and fibrosis created by HA filler can endure as long as those created by the Latera implant.

To improve breathing, filler has been placed by the senior author in the internal valves, in the scroll, and externally along the nasal sidewalls. The internal valve placement consists of 0.1 mL placed intranasally, with a 29-gauge needle, in the space between the upper lateral cartilage and the top of the septum. The scroll placement consists of less than 0.1 mL placed endonasally, between the cephalic border of the LLC and the caudal edge of the upper lateral cartilage. Finally, external placement of 0.2 to 0.3 mL can be done for the nasal sidewalls. The recommended plane of injection is again down on the perichondrium. Patients who have received filler in these locations have reported an improvement in their breathing and appear to have reduced dynamic collapse of the nose (Video 2).

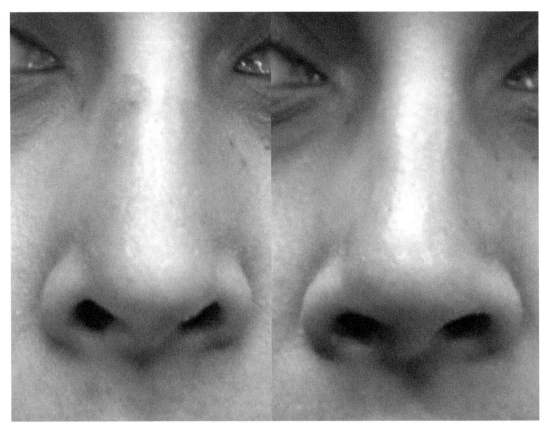

Fig. 8. Placement of 0.1 mL of HA filler along the alar rim can help correct mild cases of alar retraction and/or asymmetry. This area must be injected very slowly with frequent aspiration to reduce the risk of vascular compromise.

SUMMARY

Nonsurgical rhinoplasty is a safe and straightforward alternative to surgery for reshaping the nose. Knowledge of the vascular anatomy and proper filler choice and placement are of paramount importance. The nasal tip can be rotated and projected; dorsal height can be raised, and the nose can be straightened with filler placement in the nose.

SUPPLEMENTARY DATA

Supplementary data related to this article can be found online at https://doi.org/10.1016/j.fsc.2019.04.008.

REFERENCES

1. American Society of Plastics Surgeons. "2017 Plastic Surgery Statistics Report." 2017 Plastic Surgery Statistics, ASPS Pucblic Relations. Available at: www.plasticsurgery.org/documents/News/Statistics/2017/plastic-surgery-statistics-report-2017.pdf.
2. Daniel RK, Letourneau A. Rhinoplasty. Ann Plast Surg 1988;20(1):5–13.
3. Saban Y, Andretto Amodeo C, Bouaziz D, et al. Nasal arterial vasculature. Arch Facial Plast Surg 2012;14(6):429.
4. Toriumi DM, Mueller RA, Grosch T, et al. Vascular anatomy of the nose and the external rhinoplasty approach-reply. Arch Otolaryngol Head Neck Surg 1996;122(11):1277.
5. Jasin ME. Nonsurgical rhinoplasty using dermal fillers. Facial Plast Surg Clin North Am 2013;21(2):241–52.
6. Moon HJ. Injection rhinoplasty using filler. Facial Plast Surg Clin North Am 2018;26(3):323–30.
7. Chen Q, Liu Y, Fan D, et al. Serious vascular complications after nonsurgical rhinoplasty. Plast Reconstr Surg Glob Open 2016;4(4).
8. Urdiales-Gálvez F, Delgado NE, Figueiredo V, et al. Treatment of soft tissue filler complications: expert consensus recommendations. Aesthetic Plast Surg 2018;42(2):498–510.
9. Kim SG, Kim YJ, Lee SI, et al. Salvage of nasal skin in a case of venous compromise after hyaluronic acid filler injection using prostaglandin E. Dermatol Surg 2011;37(12):1817–9.
10. Hayreh SS. Retinal survival time and visual outcome in central retinal artery occlusion. In: Ocular vascular occlusive disorders. Springer, Cham; 2015.
11. Thanasarnaksorn W, Cotofana S, Rudolph C, et al. Severe vision loss caused by cosmetic filler augmentation: case series with review of cause and therapy. J Cosmet Dermatol 2018;17(5):712–8.
12. Kim DW, Yoon ES, Ji YH, et al. Vascular complications of hyaluronic acid fillers and the role of hyaluronidase in management. J Plast Reconstr Aesthet Surg 2011;64(12):1590–5.
13. Anderson JR. A reasoned approach to nasal base surgery. Arch Otolaryngol 1984;110(6):349–58.
14. Crumley RL, Lanser M. Quantitative analysis of nasal tip projection. Laryngoscope 1988;98(2). https://doi.org/10.1288/00005537-198802000-00017.
15. San Nicoló M, Stelter K, Sadick H, et al. Absorbable implant to treat nasal valve collapse. Facial Plast Surg 2017;33(02):233–40.

A Bioabsorbable Lateral Nasal Wall Stent for Dynamic Nasal Valve Collapse
A Review

Akshay Sanan, MD[a], Sam P. Most, MD[b,c,]*

KEYWORDS

- Nasal valve • Latera • Nasal obstruction • Lateral nasal wall • Absorbable stent

KEY POINTS

- Nasal obstruction is one of the most common clinical problems encountered by otolaryngologists and facial plastic surgeons.
- Lateral wall insufficiency (LWI) is a key anatomic contributor to nasal obstruction.
- Traditional techniques for correcting LWI include alar batten grafts, bone-anchored sutures, and lateral crural strut grafts.
- Latera is an absorbable nasal implant that can be inserted in the office or the operating room as an adjunctive procedure for LWI.

INTRODUCTION

Nasal obstruction is one of the most often encountered clinical problems treated by facial plastic surgeons. Traditionally, the most common methods for addressing nasal obstruction include septoplasty and turbinate reduction. Reconstruction of the bony-cartilaginous vault during functional rhinoplasty has addressed areas of internal nasal valve collapse.

Lateral wall insufficiency (LWI) is another anatomic contributor to nasal obstruction. The American Academy of Otolaryngology–Head & Neck Surgery recognizes multiple anatomic areas for nasal valve collapse, including those associated with LWI, and the importance of surgical correction for its repair.[1] A recent meta-analysis reviewed the efficacy of different surgical approaches to addressing LWI.[2]

Patient reported outcomes for measuring nasal obstruction are important and well-studied.[3] The most studied and validated patient reported outcome measure is the Nasal Obstruction Symptom Evaluation (NOSE) score.[4,5] A validated physician-derived grading system has been developed for zone 1 and 2 LWI, which correspond to the internal and external nasal valve, respectively (**Fig. 1**).[6] Most recently, the Standardized Cosmesis and Health Nasal Outcomes Survey (SCHNOS) scoring system has been created to further qualify nasal obstruction.[7] Together, these physician and patient grading systems of LWI and nasal obstruction provide physicians with tools to measure the efficacy of various treatments.

Disclosure Statement: Dr S.P. Most is a paid consultant of Entellus/Spirox, Inc. Dr A. Sanan has nothing to disclose.

[a] Division of Facial Plastic & Reconstructive Surgery, Stanford University School of Medicine, 801 Welch Road, Stanford, CA 94305, USA; [b] Department of Otolaryngology–Head and Neck Surgery, Stanford University School of Medicine, 801 Welch Road, Stanford, CA 94305, USA; [c] Department of Surgery (Plastic Surgery), Fellowship in Facial Plastic & Reconstructive Surgery, Division of Facial Plastic & Reconstructive Surgery, Stanford University School of Medicine, 801 Welch Road, Stanford, CA 94305, USA
* Corresponding author. 801 Welch Road, Stanford, CA 94305.
E-mail address: smost@stanford.edu

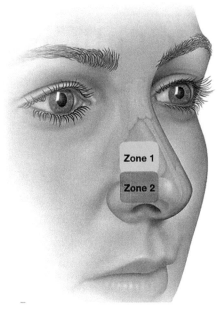

Fig. 1. Zones of lateral wall insufficiency. Zone 1 is more superior and roughly correlates to inward collapse at the level of the internal nasal valve. Zone 2 is more caudal and roughly corresponds to external nasal valve collapse. (*From* Stolovitzky P, Sidle DM, Ow RA, et al. A prospective study for treatment of nasal valve collapse due to lateral wall insufficiency: outcomes using a bioabsorbable implant. Laryngoscope 2018;128(11):2484; with permission.)

Nasal obstruction surgery is divided into 2 major types: static and dynamic. Correction of static nasal obstruction includes turbinate reduction, spreader grafts, and septoplasty (traditional and extracorporeal).[8–11] Dynamic nasal obstruction or LWI is likely caused by negative inspiratory forces being greater than the inherent strength of the lateral nasal wall, which causes inward movement.[12] The most common methods for strengthening the lateral nasal wall include batten grafts, bone-anchored sutures, and lateral crural strut grafts.[8,13–15]

The purpose of this review is to discuss Latera (Stryker, Inc, Kalamazoo, MI), a novel bioabsorbable implant to improve the nasal airway.

LATERA

The Latera nasal implant is used to support the upper and lower lateral cartilages, reinforcing the nasal wall similar to traditional cartilage grafts. It is a synthetic graft designed to withstand the negative inspiratory force and reduce LWI.

Latera Implant and Technique

The absorbable nasal implant comprises a 70:30 blend of poly(L-lactide) and poly(D-lactide). It is inserted through an endonasal insertion technique using a delivery tool. The implant is a ribbed cylindrical structure with an apical forked end (**Fig. 2**). The implant is designed to provide support to the upper and lower lateral nasal cartilages. The forked end is malleable and collapses to fit within the cannula portion of the delivery tool (**Fig. 3**). The forked end exits the delivery tool first and springs open as the implant is delivered into the tissue. The forked end is designed to anchor the implant in place.

Once delivered, the forked end is placed over the frontal process of the maxilla and the main body extends caudally toward the alar crease. The implant sits over the nasal bone and extends caudally to support the soft tissues of the area corresponding to the upper and lower lateral cartilages, thus providing strength to the lateral nasal sidewall (**Fig. 4**). The implant is flexible and easily conforms to the lateral nasal sidewall.

The implant may be placed either in the operating room in conjunction with septoplasty and/or turbinate reduction, or in the office under local anesthesia (as a stand-alone procedure or in conjunction with turbinate reduction).

Histologic Analysis of Latera

Traditionally, nonabsorbable synthetic alloplastic materials such as polyethylene, polytetrafluoroethylene, and silicone have been associated with complications including adverse tissue reaction resulting in rejection at both early and late time points. Because of this, the use of these materials has been reserved as the last choice for implantation.[16] Absorbable polymer implants such as polydioxanone and poly-lactic acid copolymers have become an option for nasal graft applications because they may reduce the postoperative complications such as extrusion (compared with permanent implants) while providing structural support as the resorbed graft material is replaced with scar tissue.[17–19]

Rippy and colleagues[20] performed a biocompatibility and absorption profile study of the Latera implant in an ovine model. The histology of the

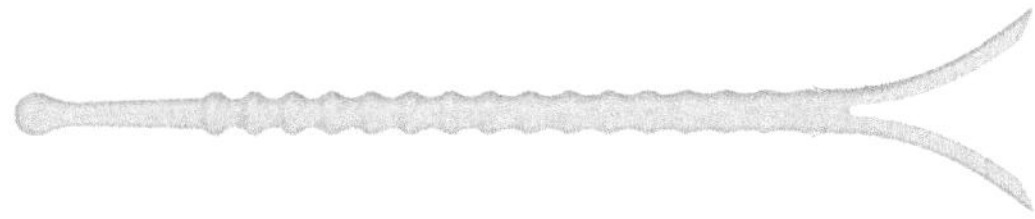

Fig. 2. Latera implant. Ribbed cylindrical structure with an apical forked end. (*Courtesy of* Stryker Inc, Kalamazoo, MI.)

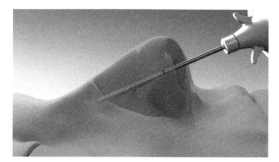

Fig. 3. Latera implant delivery device.

implant sites showed that the implants were fully encapsulated through 12 months (**Fig. 5**). The inflammatory reaction to the implants was minimal up to 12 months postprocedure. As demonstrated in histologic studies, a fibrous capsule forms and the integrity of the implant is maintained through 12 months. Tissue encapsulation promotes acute implant stability and enables localized tissue

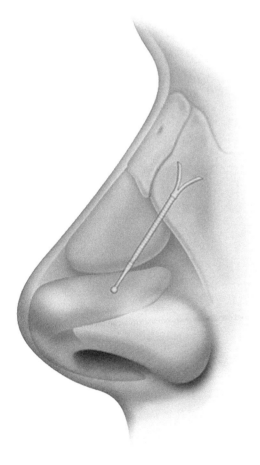

Fig. 4. Latera implant shown in proper position supporting the lateral nasal sidewall.

response during the absorption process. At 18 months, the implant material was being actively absorbed in the "mass loss" phase. By 24 months, the inflammatory reaction had diminished and complete absorption of the rod implants was noted (**Fig. 6**). Mature bundles of collagen and fibrous tissue replaced the implant, without any evidence of inflammatory tissue. The Latera implant is absorbed over a period of about 24 months.

Latera Research

The original Latera implant study by San Nicolo and colleagues[17] was a prospective 30-patient clinical trial to evaluate the safety and effectiveness of the implant for lateral wall support in nasal valve collapse in Germany. Enrolled subjects had isolated nasal valve collapse without any anatomic contributors to their nasal obstruction and a NOSE score >55. Fifty-six implants were placed in 30 subjects and assessments were made up to 12 months postprocedure. At 12 months follow-up, there was an average NOSE score reduction of 40.9 ± 31.2 points. Seventy-six percent of patients were considered responders, meaning they had at least 1 NOSE score improvement or a NOSE score reduction of at least 20%. There were no cosmetic changes or complaints at 12 months follow-up.

This study was followed up with a 24-month follow-up study by the same group.[21] The average NOSE score reduction was 44.0 ± 31.1 points. There were no device-related adverse events or cosmetic changes in the 12- to 24-month interval.

A recent study by Stolovitzky and colleagues[22] sought to examine the effectiveness and safety of Latera either alone or in combination with conventional adjunctive procedures used to open the nasal airway (septoplasty ± turbinate reduction) in the United States. Follow-up for this cohort was 6 months and the study demonstrated significant reduction in NOSE scores at this time interval. Further, a blinded physician-derived evaluation of lateral nasal wall movement, based on the LWI scale, demonstrated a significant reduction in lateral wall medialization with inhalation. These 2 independent measures, which both improved after treatment, provide evidence for the efficacy of the implant in improving the nasal airway in patients with LWI.

Latera, although safe overall, does have the risk of complications. Practitioners must counsel their patients on the possibility of implant extrusion.[17,21,22] The implants are typically retrieved by the surgeon during a follow-up visit in office following direct visualization of the implant

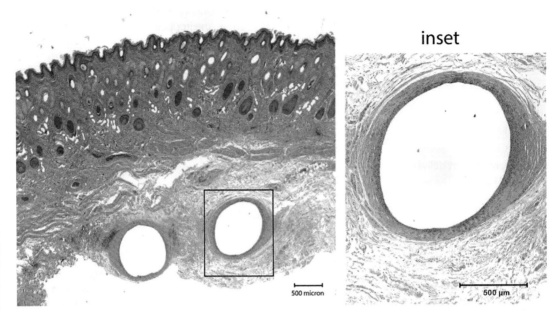

Fig. 5. Histology of implantation at 12 months. Clear round spaces correspond to implant. Implant sites do not have any inflammatory infiltrate. Capsule surrounding implant composed of macrophages and giant cells. (*From* Rippy MK, Baron S, Rosenthal M, et al. Evaluation of absorbable PLA nasal implants in an ovine model. Laryngoscope Investig Otolaryngol 2018;3(3):158; with permission.)

exposed at the endonasal cannula insertion point. Factors contributing to implant extrusion include insertion of implant too proximal to the insertion point or excessive manipulation of implant by patient. Other complications described include inflammation and infection at the surgical site, which resolved with antibiotics.

SUMMARY

As with any procedure, proper patient selection is paramount. This implant, much like most lateral nasal wall procedures, stabilizes rather than widens the nasal airway. When examining patients with nasal valve collapse, it is important to

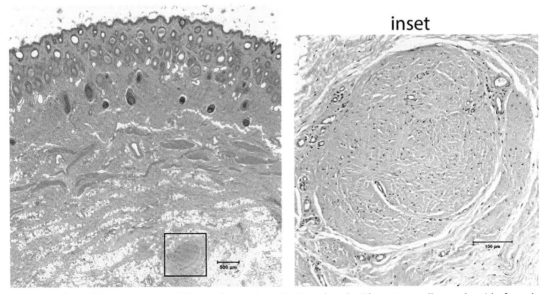

Fig. 6. Histology of implantation at 24 months. Implant site is replaced with mature collagen devoid of any inflammatory cells or implant. (*From* Rippy MK, Baron S, Rosenthal M, et al. Evaluation of absorbable PLA nasal implants in an ovine model. Laryngoscope Investig Otolaryngol 2018;3(3):159; with permission.)

determine if there is any LWI. If nasal obstructive symptoms during inhalation are improved with stabilization (not lateralization) of the nasal sidewall, the patient may be a candidate for this implant. Only in these cases would stabilization of the nasal wall with a Latera implant improve nasal obstructive symptoms. Twenty-four-month postoperative data demonstrate the safety and efficacy of this novel treatment. Latera is a safe procedure that can be done under local anesthesia. More long-term studies need to demonstrate its efficacy, and ideally a randomized placebo control study should be performed.

REFERENCES

1. Rhee JS, Weaver EM, Park SS, et al. Clinical consensus statement: diagnosis and management of nasal valve compromise. Otolaryngol Head Neck Surg 2010;143:48–59.
2. Kandathil CK, Spataro EA, Laimi K, et al. Repair of the lateral nasal wall in nasal airway obstruction: a meta-analysis. JAMA Facial Plast Surg 2018. https://doi.org/10.1001/jamafa- cial.2018.0036.
3. Lam DJ, James KT, Weaver EM. Comparison of anatomic, physiological, and subjective measures of the nasal airway. Am J Rhinol 2006;20:463–70.
4. Stewart MG, Witsell DL, Smith TL, et al. Development and validation of the Nasal Obstruction Symptom Evaluation (NOSE) scale. Otolaryngol Head Neck Surg 2004;130:157–63.
5. Stewart MG, Smith TL, Weaver EM, et al. Outcomes after nasal septoplasty: results from the Nasal Obstruction Septoplasty Effectiveness (NOSE) study. Otolaryngol Head Neck Surg 2004;130: 283–90.
6. Tsao GJ, Fijalkowski N, Most SP. Validation of a grading system for lateral nasal wall insufficiency. Allergy Rhinol (Providence) 2013;4:e66–8.
7. Moubayed SP, Ionnaidis JPA, Saltychev M, et al. The 10-item standardized cosmesis and health nasal outcomes survey (SCHNOS) for functional and cosmetic rhinoplasty. JAMA Facial Plast Surg 2018;20(1):37–42.
8. Goode RL. Surgery of the incompetent nasal valve. Laryngoscope 1985;95:546–55.
9. Most SP. Anterior septal reconstruction: outcomes after a modified extra-corporeal septoplasty technique. Arch Facial Plast Surg 2006;8:202–7.
10. Sheen JH. Spreader graft: a method of reconstructing the roof of the middle nasal vault following rhinoplasty. Plast Reconstr Surg 1984;73:230–9.
11. Surowitz J, Lee MK, Most SP. Anterior septal reconstruction for treatment of severe caudal septal deviation: clinical severity and outcomes. Otolaryngol Head Neck Surg 2015;153:27–33.
12. Keeler J, Most SP. Measuring nasal obstruction. Facial Plast Surg Clin North Am 2016;24:315–22.
13. Vaezeafshar R, Moubayed SP, Most SP. Repair of lateral wall insufficiency. JAMA Facial Plast Surg 2018;20:111–5.
14. Roofe SB, Most SP. Placement of a lateral nasal suspension suture via an external rhinoplasty approach. Arch Facial Plast Surg 2007;9:214–6.
15. Paniello RC. Nasal valve suspension. An effective treatment for nasal valve collapse. Arch Otolaryngol Head Neck Surg 1996;122:1342–6.
16. Lovice DB, Mingrone MD, Toriumi DM. Grafts and implants in rhinoplasty and nasal reconstruction. Otolaryngol Clin North Am 1999;32(1):113–41.
17. San Nicolo M, Stelter K, Sadick H, et al. Absorbable implant to treat nasal valve collapse. Facial Plast Surg 2017;33:233–40.
18. Boenisch M, Mink A. Clinical and histological results of septoplasty with a resorbable implant. Arch Otolaryngol Head Neck Surg 2000;126(11):1373–7.
19. Della Santina CC, Byrne PJ. Initial management of total nasal septectomy defects using resorbable plating. Arch Facial Plast Surg 2013;8(2):128–38.
20. Rippy MK, Baron S, Rosenthal M, et al. Evaluation of absorbable PLA nasal implants in an ovine model. Laryngoscope Investig Otolaryngol 2018;3(3): 156–61.
21. San Nicolo M, Stelter K, Sadick H, et al. A 2-year follow-up study of an absorbable implant to treat nasal valve collapse. Facial Plast Surg 2018;34:1–6.
22. Stolovitzky P, Sidle DM, Ow RA, et al. A prospective study for treatment of nasal valve collapse due to lateral wall insufficiency: outcomes using a bioabsorbable implant. Laryngoscope 2018. https://doi.org/10.1002/lary.27242.

Social Media Marketing in Facial Plastic Surgery
What Has Worked?

Laxmeesh Mike Nayak, MD[a],*, Gary Linkov, MD[b]

KEYWORDS

- Social media • Marketing • Facial plastics • Instagram • Facebook • Snapchat

KEY POINTS

- Social media is quickly becoming one of the main avenues for direct to consumer marketing.
- Patients use social media to find surgeons and to communicate about procedures, outcomes, and their experiences.
- A surgeon's social media presence can dramatically increase their perception of being an expert and showcase to patients their style and approach.
- There is no single best social network, instead various networks exist with unique characteristics that each have the potential to drive traffic to a practice.
- Social media can be potentially hazardous for patients and surgeons if misused.

INTRODUCTION

As patients incorporate social media into their daily routine, physicians are increasingly investigating ways of harnessing this burgeoning market of interactive media. Plastic surgeons are apt to embrace innovation and emerging technologies, and they are now helping to define the interaction between social media and medicine. Social media is a powerful tool that needs to be used wisely to avoid pitfalls.

SOCIAL MEDIA

Social media is an opportunity for people to connect electronically and informally. It is designed to make introductions, share experiences, build community, and overall link people with common interests.[1] Social media platforms represent a dynamic and powerful tool to educate, engage, market to, and directly communicate with patients and professional colleagues.[2] It can include chat rooms, blogs, networks, or channels. In the very intimate world of plastic surgery, it offers an opportunity to interact and learn more in greater dimension than traditional media, yet social media still allows patients to remain anonymous, if they so choose.[1] Most forms of social media function as a freemium business model, whereby the use of basic services is free but certain promotional features come with a price tag.

There are several different kinds of social media (discussed below).

Networks

Social networks, such as Facebook, Twitter, Instagram, and Snapchat, include services whereby personal or business accounts are created and "friends" or "followers" connect. Instagram and Snapchat are primarily used on mobile devices and consist mainly of photographs and video content. Other networks, such as LinkedIn, are for professional networking as a way to connect with business contacts.

Disclosure Statement: The authors have nothing to disclose.
[a] Nayak Plastic Surgery, 607 South Lindbergh Boulevard, St Louis, MO 63131, USA; [b] City Facial Plastics, 635 Madison Avenue #407, New York, NY 10065, USA
* Corresponding author.
E-mail address: mikenayak@gmail.com

Facial Plast Surg Clin N Am 27 (2019) 373–377
https://doi.org/10.1016/j.fsc.2019.04.002

Forums

The original chat room forums such as AOL have been replaced by more sophisticated Web sites such as Reddit, which has many "subreddits" that unite individuals with similar, targeted interests and create a framework for discussion and promotion of interesting content.

Video Sharing

YouTube and Vimeo offer robust video sharing capability with potential to handle longer educational content and store it in a more permanent fashion. Instagram and Snapchat also offer video content sharing with shorter videos that are often only temporarily available to the user's network.

Reviews

Historically, review sites were meant more for restaurants and movies, but now physicians have a lot to gain or lose based on their reviews. Sites such as Healthgrades offer little conversation between the patient and physician, and are primarily a 1-way exchange for patients to post about their experience. Other review sites such as RealSelf, Yelp, and Google allow for practices to at least respond to patient reviews, although in a limited capacity because of HIPAA regulations.

HOW WE USE IT

Several studies in the plastic surgery literature have sought to investigate how we currently use social media. The first study, in 2013, found that the reasons for using social media, namely Facebook, included the beliefs that incorporation of social media into medical practice is inevitable (56.7%), that they are an effective marketing tool (52.1%), and that they provide a forum for patient education (49%). Surgeons with a primarily esthetic surgery practice were more likely to use social media.[2]

Chang and colleagues[3] found that plastic surgeons using Facebook are younger compared with nonusers. They also found that users and nonusers believe the greatest benefits of Facebook are increased practice exposure and low-cost advertising; however, seldom are objective outcomes tracked. Facebook users were therefore encouraged to monitor its direct effects on quantifiable outcomes, such as professional Web site traffic, number of new patient referrals, conversion-to-surgery rates, and operative volume, to clarify whether or not its continued use is worth the effort.

AUTHORS' IMPRESSIONS OF MAJOR PLATFORMS AS THEY APPLY TO FACIAL PLASTIC SURGERY

Facebook's demographic tends to encompass adults from their mid to late 20s through to senior citizens. This platform also allows for multiple pictures per post, videos over an hour long, and detailed text descriptions. For these reasons, education-heavy, explanatory posts, or posts about surgical and nonsurgical antiaging interventions, may be fit more naturally on Facebook than other current platforms.

Snapchat, in contrast, is the most spontaneous, least formal of all current platforms, with a core demographic ranging from preteens to late 30s. Owing to the design of the application, users can predominately only post sequential video clips in a sequential, minimally processed manner. It is really not practical to post significant text, curated photos, or heavily produced video. Most Snapchat "stories" sunset automatically in 24 hours, and may not be viewed on the poster's account after that point. Most adults have heard at least this 1 fact of Snapchat, and are often more willing to share their surgical footage or results on that platform for that reason.

Video clips are generally posted from a first-person point of view, in real time. Snapchat stories feel authentic because they are minimally produced. Snapchat's primary value, then, over other platforms, is its ability to give the viewers a feeling of knowing the poster more personally. It is not uncommon for Snapchat followers to "feel like they already know" their surgeon before they have ever met.

Instagram's demographic, similarly, runs from preteens through late 30s. Being an inherently visual platform, Instagram lends itself very well to a profile full of carefully curated before and after photos, each with a relatively small amount of descriptive text. Short video segments of 59 seconds or less may also be posted. Hashtag indexing of posts tends to be more important on Instagram, as many users search for and follow not just individual accounts, but new posts on hashtag subjects of interest.

Instagram's recently introduced "stories" feature is essentially a Snapchat clone, and carries similar strength and limitations as described above. Well-managed Instagram accounts can leverage interplay between their enduring Instagram posts and ephemeral stories to further influence their followers. With the introduction of Instagram stories, speculation has grown that Snapchat will continue to lose relevance to Instagram.

YouTube is designed and built for video sharing, with no still photos and minimal caption text. YouTube videos may range from seconds to hours, and may be streamed in several formats, from smartphone-compatible to ultra-high resolution. Videos can also be tagged with keywords to ensure they are served automatically to viewers with matching interests. Because of these strengths, YouTube is the best platform for hosting and sharing detailed videos with semiprofessional or even professional production values (**Table 1**)

WHAT PATIENTS WANT

Asking patients about their favorite networks and their preferred type of content may help improve a plastic surgeon's success in building a practice through social media. In 2017, Sorice and colleagues[4] found that Facebook and Instagram were the only 2 networks used several times a day by over 10% of patients surveyed. Despite the importance of social media, patients stated that the practice Web site was the most important online platform that influenced their decision to choose the practice. When asked about which Web site content was most important to patients, the leading factor was before and after photographs followed by information about procedures.

IS IT WORTH IT?

A recent publication from 2018 by Gould and Nazarian,[5] adopted a business model called the 3-M framework for understanding social media and customer dialogue originally developed for Starbucks, and applied it to plastic surgery. In it, the elements include the megaphone (surgeon to patient), magnet (patient to surgeon), and monitor (patient to patient and surgeon to surgeon). They found a consistent trend of growth associated with all social media sources over time, contrasted with the flat or downtrending return on investment with a practice Web site, Google, and Yelp. Importantly, word of mouth was seen as having the largest potential for growth, and reinvesting in the existing patient base was emphasized. The authors concluded that social media and branding campaigns for start-up practices, using Instagram and direct to consumer marketing, followed by Yelp, RealSelf, Facebook, and Google SEO for maintenance of the early practice, and then strategic investment in the patient base once established to bootstrap and leverage the word of mouth referrals.

#HASHTAG

Twitter and Instagram encourages the use of hashtags to make content more discoverable. Using the hashtag as a method to better curate content online may allow lay audiences to better identify quality information. Members of the Urology, Radiology, Oncology, and Gastroenterology specialties have devised hashtag ontologies that seek to unify all hashtags and organize discussion on specific medical topics. Hashtags may help drive dialogue among informed individuals and groups while filtering out "noise" posted by individuals not purposefully intending to join the scientific and clinical discussion.[6] Facial plastic surgeons should seek a more active role in organizing social media dialogue by devising a hashtag ontology. Although patients may use certain lay terms, surgeons have the potential to organize information in more accurate and consistent terms that set apart the specialists from those pretending to be specialists.

POTENTIAL PITFALLS
Time Investment

Today's practice environment puts many demands on our time. We should continue to assess the value of social media, especially given its ability to consume a significant percentage of our time and effort. The larger our social media accounts become, the more demanding our followers are for fresh and frequent content.

Table 1
Select social media platforms with highlights of their demographics, format, and advantages

Platform	Facebook	Snapchat	Instagram	YouTube
Demographics	Mid 20s and up	Preteen-30s	Preteen-30s	Teens and up
Format	Photo; video	Video	Photo; video	Video
Advantages	• Education • Antiaging	• Videos sunset in 24 h • Real-time authenticity	• Curated content • Hashtag indexing	• Detailed videos • High-resolution streaming

Ethical and Legal Concerns

To maintain the respect of medical peers and the public, it is critical for facial plastic surgeons to use social media to provide factual information regarding surgery while protecting patient identity and professionally caring for the patient population.[7]

It is important to remember that data placed on the internet may not be easy to remove if and when a patient chooses to no longer be featured on our social media feeds.

Unwanted Solicitations from Advertisers

Advertisers often promise practices, especially on Instagram, swarms of new followers and promotion with little or no evidence or description that their service will be effective or legal. Increasing a follower base by hiring companies that use bots to artificially inflate your numbers is a recipe for getting removed from the network, or eventually seeing a drastic decline in followers after the bots are removed by the network. The best and most authentic way to grow a following is to post consistently relevant and informative material that potential patients find useful and relatable.

Negative Comments

Creating and maintaining a presence on social media has the potential to expose a practice to negative comments, either on review sites or media-sharing sites. These comments can be damaging as they are perpetually visible to potential patients, and often surgeons have no recourse due to privacy matters.

Unrealistic Expectations

Although patients may become more informed in some aspects through various posted photos and videos, they may also develop unrealistic and potentially dangerous overall expectations. Patients may come to expect a certain result after seeing it online without realizing that their particular situation may be unique and might alter the end result.

Experts Versus Amateurs

Competition between social media accounts occurs on an uneven playing field. For instance, ethical, expert providers will take care to standardize before and after photo lighting and positioning, and truthfully depict the time, cost, and risk involved in recovery. Amateur providers, however, may not realize that a "before" photo with heavy shadows and overhead lighting, paired with an "after" photo with strong front flash or softbox light effect, is misleading and shows a greater improvement than matched photos would. These misleading "improvements" created by lighting, head position, or makeup may not be intentional, but the public can be misled into thinking the results are real.

Education and Experience Versus Follower Count

In the past, consumers used board certification, years in practice, and in-person word of mouth as proxies for a practice's standing or reputability. In the current social media era, for better or worse, follower counts and online celebrity are replacing those other measures.

Personal Versus Professional

As facial plastic surgeons begin to expose their practices to the community at large using modern social media tools, often aspects of their personal life will bleed into their professional life. To what degree are we jeopardizing our families and loved ones or blurring the distinction between doctor and friend to our patients. These are issues we must all grapple with in our social media era.

SUMMARY

Social media are quickly becoming one of the main avenues for direct to consumer marketing. Patients use social media to find surgeons and to communicate about procedures, outcomes, and their experiences. A surgeon's social media presence can dramatically increase their perception of being an expert and showcase to patients their style and approach. There is no single best social network, instead various networks exist with unique characteristics that each have the potential to drive traffic to a practice. Social media can be potentially hazardous for patients and surgeons if misused.

REFERENCES

1. Kuechel MC. Showcase your service: social media and marketing basics in a dynamic, over-populated, mixed-message, and highly competitive world. Facial Plast Surg Clin North Am 2010;18(4):533–6.
2. Vardanian AJ, Kusnezov N, Im DD, et al. Social media use and impact on plastic surgery practice. Plast Reconstr Surg 2013;131(5):1184–93.
3. Chang JB, Woo SL, Cederna PS. Worth the "likes"? The use of facebook among plastic surgeons and its perceived impact. Plast Reconstr Surg 2015; 135(5):909e–18e.

4. Sorice SC, Li AY, Gilstrap J, et al. Social media and the plastic surgery patient. Plast Reconstr Surg 2017;140(5):1047–56.

5. Gould DJ, Nazarian S. Social media return on investment: how much is it worth to my practice? Aesthet Surg J 2018;38(5):565–74.

6. Chiang AL, Vartabedian B, Spiegel B. Harnessing the hashtag: a standard approach to GI dialogue on social media. Am J Gastroenterol 2016;111(8):1082–4.

7. Gutierrez PL, Johnson DJ. Can plastic surgeons maintain professionalism within social media? AMA J Ethics 2018;20(4):379–83.

What's New in Facial Hair Transplantation?
Effective Techniques for Beard and Eyebrow Transplantation

Anthony Bared, MD*

KEYWORDS

- Facial hair transplantation • Hair restoration • Beard transplantation • Eyebrow transplantation
- Follicular unit extraction (FUE) • No-shave follicular unit extraction

KEY POINTS

- Advances in hair transplantation techniques allow natural results in facial hair transplantation to be achieved.
- Poor hair growth angulation can occur occasionally despite the best efforts in acute recipient site angulation and hair placement.
- Eyebrows will start to regrow around 4 to 6 months after transplant and will continue to fill in for a full year, gradually increasing in density.

INTRODUCTION

Advances in hair restoration techniques have made it possible to transplant hair in nonscalp areas of the face such as the beard and eyebrows. Refinements in techniques have allowed for the transplantation of beard hair and eyebrow hair with natural appearing results. Thick eyebrows and full beards are in vogue. Pick up any of the latest fashion magazines and you see female models with thick, full eyebrows, or men sporting beards. Our practice has seen a large increase in the demand for beard and eyebrow transplantation. This article describes the preoperative consultation, operative technique, and postoperative care developed from our experience of over 1000 procedures in facial hair restoration.

BEARD TRANSPLANTATION
Preoperative Planning

Most patients seeking facial hair restoration are men with a genetic paucity of facial hair (**Fig. 1**).

Other reasons for patients seeking facial hair restoration are for poorly thought out previous laser hair removal, scarring, burn, or cleft lip repair (**Fig. 2**). Another small group are female to male transgender patients seeking a more masculine appearance. Treatment goals in beard restoration are often set by the patient. Patients typically present with a rather specific understanding of how they want their facial hair to appear. A patient's goals may vary from increasing the density of an existing beard while maintaining the same shape, to transplanting full beards where few hairs exist. The design and density of the beard may be limited by the quality and quantity of the donor area. Transplantation of full beards requires a large amount of grafts and patients are always made aware of the possibility of undergoing secondary procedures after 1 year if further density is desired. These grafts, it must be made clear, once transplanted, will no longer be available for use in the scalp in the future if male pattern hair loss is to develop.

Disclosure Statement: The author has nothing to disclose.
Private Practice, Miami, FL, USA
* 6280 Sunset Drive, Suite 504, Miami, FL 33143.
E-mail address: abared@dranthonybared.com

Facial Plast Surg Clin N Am 27 (2019) 379–384
https://doi.org/10.1016/j.fsc.2019.04.003
1064-7406/19/© 2019 Published by Elsevier Inc.

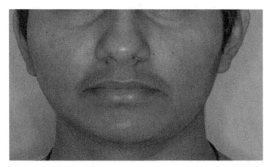

Fig. 1. Male patient with a paucity of facial hair presenting for beard hair transplantation.

With the advances and refinements in follicular unit extraction (FUE) techniques, most patients seen in our office elect to have the procedure performed in this manner to avoid a linear scar, allowing them to maintain a short hairstyle.[1,2] FUE has largely replaced the traditional strip donor extractions for beard transplantation in our office.[3,4] Regardless of the donor technique used, patients are made aware of the potential limitations of the donor hair quantity and therefore "size" and density of the beard that can be achieved through a single procedure. It is our experience that the scalp hair transplants to the face have a high regrowth percentage and, if properly performed, patients can achieve a natural outcome. As in any cosmetic procedure, listening to the patient's exact goals and desires is imperative. Patients who desire facial hair restorations, in general, express a specific desire for how they want their beard designed. Depending on the exact design and density, graft counts can range from 250 to 300 grafts to each sideburn, 400 to 800 grafts to the mustache and goatee, and 300 to 500 grafts per cheek. These numbers can vary based on the pre-existing hair, design, and thickness of the donor hair.

As with other hair transplantation cases, patients need to be in good general health and off medications, supplements, and vitamins that can worsen bleeding.

Surgical Preparation

As mentioned, most patients have a specific idea about the design they wish for their facial hair. Using the patient's guidelines, the areas to be transplanted are marked out using a surgical marking pen with the patient in a seated position. The markings are checked for symmetry between the 2 sides. Measurements are used to help ensure symmetry. Patients are shown the markings in a mirror, in case the 2-dimensional perspective provided by a mirror—which is what the patient sees in a mirror—is different than what the surgeon sees in direct three dimensions. If then needed, alterations are made according to patient desires (**Fig. 3**).

Procedural Approach

Currently in our practice, the vast majority of patients seeking facial hair restoration elect to have their procedure using the FUE technique to avoid a linear scar. In these cases, the donor area is usually shaved (a no-shave FUE alternative is also offered), and the patient is placed in a supine position. The donor area is prepped and draped in a sterile fashion for the procedure. Local anesthesia is infiltrated into the donor area. The smallest possible drill size avoiding graft transection is used for the extractions. The donor area consists of the occiput only in smaller cases and extends into the parietal scalp for larger cases. Graft extractions are evenly distributed throughout the donor area to avoid areas of focal alopecia. Once the extractions have been completed from the occipital area, the patient is then turned to lie in the supine position.

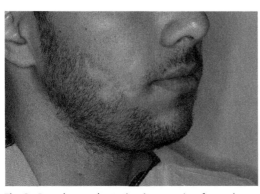

Fig. 2. Beard transplantation is an option for male patients to help camouflage facial scars.

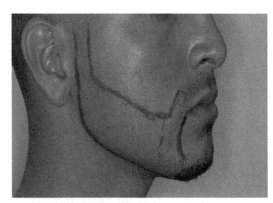

Fig. 3. Patients are marked in the preoperative suite before facial hair transplantation where they are shown the outline and design of the beard.

Local anesthesia is then applied to the face starting in each sideburn and cheek area. The area around the mouth is not anesthetized at this point; the area around the mouth is typically worked on after the patient has eaten lunch. The recipient sites in the sideburn and cheek area are made first. The smallest possible recipient sites are made using 0.5-, 0.6-, or 0.7-mm slits. The 1, 2, and (if used) 3 hair grafts are tested to ensure size compatibility with the recipient sites. In the periphery of the sideburns, 1 hair graft is used whereas 2 hair grafts can be placed in the central aspect of the sideburn to allow for more density (**Fig. 4**). Counter traction is provided by the nondominant hand and an assistant while making the incisions. The key esthetic step is to make the incisions at an ultra-acute angle to the skin, with the direction of the incisions determined by either existing surrounding hairs or the fine "peach fuzz" of the face. This being said, the direction of growth is generally downward, but more centrally closer to the mouth/goatee region can be somewhat anterior. In the cheek area, 3 hair grafts are sometimes used in the central beard in patients with finer hair to allow for the achievement of greater density without a compromise of naturalness. If further grafts are needed, they are extracted at this time from the parietal scalp. The patient's head is slightly turned, allowing for the simultaneous extraction of grafts from the parietal area and the placement of grafts in the ipsilateral cheek and sideburn.

After the patient is given lunch, the area around the mouth is then anesthetized. Infraorbital and mental nerve blocks are used to provide initial anesthesia. Anesthesia in the goatee and mustache area is then reinforced with field subdermal local anesthesia complemented by epinephrine 1:60,000 to minimize bleeding. Incisions in the goatee and mustache area are then made. On the mustache, hairs will grow slightly laterally

and then transition downward along the goatee. Patients need to be made aware of the difficulty in creating density along the entire mustache, particularly centrally within the "Cupid's bow." The creation of density in this area is difficult owing to the undulations created by the upper lip's Cupid's bow area. It is also important to maintain as acute an angle as possible in this central area of the upper lip because grafts have a tendency to grow straight outward in nonacute angles. The transition from the mustache to the goatee is an important area for the creation of density, which is usually created by the maximal dense packing of 2 hair grafts.

The grafts are placed into these recipient sites using jeweler's forceps. Counter traction splaying the incision sites open with the nondominant hand helps in the placement of the grafts given the laxity of facial skin. The importance of having experienced assistants for this process is critical, as they need to understand the "pattern" of graft distribution, as created by the surgeon. Toward the conclusion of the procedure, the patient is given a mirror before all grafts are placed. Given that the immediate results closely replicate the final results, it is helpful for the patient to view their beard to assess the design and density of the grafts. This allows for feedback, fine-tuning, and alteration before the conclusion of the procedure (**Fig. 5**).

Postprocedure Care

Patients are told to keep their face dry for the first 5 days after the procedure. This allows for the grafts to set properly, helping to assure the maintenance of proper angulation. Topical antibiotic ointment is applied to the donor area. Patients are then to wet their face with soap and water,

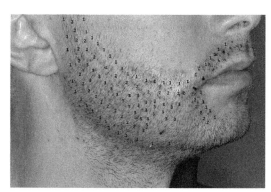

Fig. 4. Image demonstrating the typical graft size placement for beard transplantation.

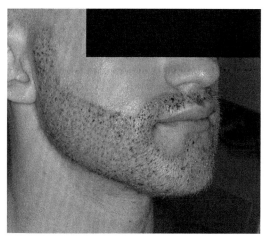

Fig. 5. Immediate postopereative results where patients are able to see their beard design.

starting to remove the dried blood and crusts. Shaving is permitted after 10 days. Hair regrowth usually starts around 4 to 6 months. The transplanted hair can be treated as any other facial hair and allowed to grow out or shaved. Most patients are satisfied with the initial density from 1 procedure but a secondary, touch-up procedure, can be performed after 1 year to create further density.

Potential Complications and Their Management

Poor angulation

Hairs can grow out perpendicularly giving the beard an unnatural appearance. As previously mentioned, the area of the face where improper angulation poses the greatest challenge is in the mustache. To avoid the improper angulation it is helpful to use the smallest possible incision at an acute angle. It is helpful to use a longer blade so as to allow it to lay flat across the skin permitting a sharply acute angle. If needed, the perpendicular hair grafts can be removed via the FUE technique and the resulting hole is left to heal by secondary intention.

Bump formation

Tiny bumps can form, particularly under the lip in the "soul patch" and chin mound areas at the site of the transplanted grafts. The cause of the formation of these bumps is not known; however, this is mostly seen in patients with thick, dark hair. As the hair grows in this soul patch and chin mound area, a small bump can form where the hair exits the skin. For this reason, if a patient desires hair in these regions, a small "test" procedure can be performed at the time of the initial procedure, or alternatively, only single-hair grafts trimmed of surrounding skin can be used safely. If, in 6 to 8 months, no bumps have formed then further hair can be transplanted.[5] Patients of Asian ethnicity, particularly those with dark thick hairs, are the most challenging on whom to avoid complications, both in this bump formation, but also in achieving naturalness owing to the difficulty in getting the grafts to look natural, particularly in angulation. With these Asian patients, the less-experienced surgeon is strongly encouraged to proceed conservatively, with the primary use of all single-hair grafts and a smaller number of grafts, until proficiency is achieved.

EYEBROW TRANSPLANTATION
Preoperative Planning

The goal in eyebrow restoration is to restore the desired shape and density, and natural direction and angle of growth of eyebrow hair. The most common presentation in women is the thinning of the eyebrows, either from over-plucking, aging, or genetic causes. In cases of complete eyebrow absence, types of alopecia (such as alopecia totalis) need to be ruled out before considering transplantation.[6] Men typically lose the lateral aspect of the eyebrows with aging and are seeking overall thicker eyebrows. Some of our female patients have had previous permanent makeup, and are advised that this may compromise regrowth in the occasional case. These tattoos can often help guide the design of the eyebrows, but oftentimes we find that they were made asymmetrically and/or not esthetically. Most of our female patients are able to draw their desired eyebrows, which we encourage, but then often require some fine-tuning by the surgeon to create a nicer look.

The donor hair is almost always the scalp because of its reliable regrowth, although other areas of the body can be used as well, but the regrowth is not as reliable, nor is supply often readily available. In most cases, scalp donor hair extraction is performed from a small "strip" from the occipital scalp. The strip technique allows for the hair to be maintained slightly longer as it exits the skin, allowing for the visualization of the direction of growth of the hair. In some cases, particularly in men, the FUE technique is used. Overall, given the small number of grafts needed, patients are given the option of the "no-shave" FUE technique so that they can avoid the trimming of the donor area and maintain their hair longer.

Surgical Preparation

Patients are seated in front of a mirror in the preoperative suite. Women generally have a good idea of the shape they desire for their eyebrows. They are asked to bring in photos of "model" eyebrows to help guide their design. After preoperative photos are obtained, if the patient has a good idea of the shape they desire, they are offered an eye-liner pen and are given the time to draw in their desired eyebrow shape. The patient's active involvement in the design of their eyebrows is important. After they are given some time to design their eyebrows, final markings and refinements are made by the surgeon with a semipermanent fine marker. Measurements are taken for symmetry. Men seeking eyebrow restoration typically are seeking to fill in areas within the eyebrows that are lacking density. The male eyebrow is designed with less of an arch and as an extension of the existing eyebrow. Photos are obtained after the final markings have been made.

The author likes to divide the eyebrow into 3 sections:

1. Head (innermost 5–8 mm)
2. Body (central 2.5–3.5 cm)
3. Tail (outer 2–2.5 cm)

In women, the point at which the tail and body meet forming the arch is usually located at or just lateral to the lateral limbus of the eye. For a more dramatic look, this arch can be as far lateral to the lateral canthal region. However, it can vary in position and roundedness. In men, the arch of the brow is not so much as a peek but rather a widening of the eyebrow along the area correlating to the lateral limbus. This is best demonstrated in **Fig. 6**.

Procedural Approach

If a strip harvesting technique is to be used, the patient remains in the upright, seated position for the excision. The strip is typically harvested from the occipital scalp and, depending on the number of grafts needed, varies in length and width from about 3 to 5 cm and 10 to 15 mm, respectively. If the FUE technique is used, the patient is placed in the prone position for donor harvesting. Given the smaller number of grafts needed, shaving of the entire donor area can be avoided. Once the donor hairs have been harvested the patient is then positioned in a supine "beach chair" position for incision site placement. Highly experienced technicians perform the dissection of the harvested donor hairs under the microscope, under the supervision of the surgeon. Naturally occurring 1- and 2-hair follicular units are dissected, although, in some cases, 3 hair follicular units are used to achieve maximal density without compromising naturalness.

The eyebrows are anesthetized, and 1:50,000 epinephrine is injected for hemostasis. Recipient sites are created by the surgeon using the smallest blade size appropriate for the grafts, most commonly 0.5 mm, but sometimes 0.6 mm for the occasional larger 2 hair grafts and even 3 hair grafts. Recipient sites are first made along the boundaries of the eyebrow along the preoperative markings, as these markings can be lost with the subsequent bleeding and wiping of the blood from the recipient sites. Paying attention to the proper direction of growth is critical. Within the head of the eyebrow, hair usually grows in a more vertical/superior direction. Moving from the more inferior to the more superior aspect of the head of the brow the hairs quickly change direction to grow in a more horizontal then inferior/downward direction, particularly along the superior border. Moving laterally, the hairs along the superior border are oriented in an inferior/downward direction, while the hairs along the inferior border are oriented in a superior/upward direction, creating a herring-bone pattern (**Fig. 7**). This cross-hatching continues throughout the body of the eyebrow until the tail portion, where the hairs then are primarily oriented horizontally. Incisions are made as flat (acute an angle) as possible to the skin (**Fig. 8**). Once all the recipient sites are made bilaterally, the grafts are then inserted. Care is taken to orient the hairs so that the direction of growth (ie, the curl) of the hair is in an acute angle with the skin. We like to place as many 2-hair grafts as possible, except along the innermost head and lateralmost tail portion, where 1-hair grafts are used. If 3-hair grafts are deemed appropriate, they are placed in the central aspect of the body portion, to achieve maximal density. It is critical to make just about all of the recipient sites before any planting is to be done, then, after all these recipient sites are filled with grafts, the patient is asked to sit up and the eyebrows are inspected; small adjustments can then be made with the placement of more grafts. The patient can then view the eyebrows to obtain his/her feedback regarding symmetry and the desired shape.

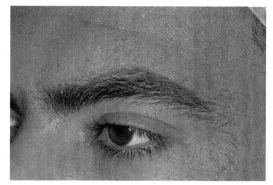

Fig. 6. Male eyebrow demonstrating the lateral thickening over the area of the lateral limbus.

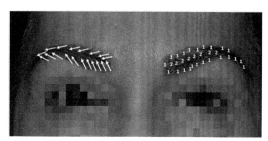

Fig. 7. Image demonstrating the direction of eyebrow graft placement and the size of the grafts.

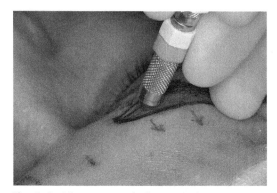

Fig. 8. Incisions are made in an angle as acute as possible to the skin.

Potential Complications and Their Management

The most common complications related to eyebrow hair restorations are asymmetry, rather than anticipated hair regrowth, and poor hair angulation. It is important when marking the eyebrows that symmetry is checked and rechecked. It is also helpful to view the immediate photo once the markings have been made. The viewing of the photos helps to provide a "third" eye and different perspective, often revealing asymmetries that may not have been immediately apparent. As mentioned previously, recipient sites are first made along these markings, along the boundaries of the eyebrow, before they can be rubbed off and lost. The local anesthesia and the swelling can create asymmetries during the procedure, making 1 eyebrow appear higher than the other and thus creating artifactual asymmetric appearances that are more difficult to correct at the end of the procedure. To limit this phenomenon, it is best to administer the local anesthetic at the beginning of the case and to have the patient sit up to check for symmetry before adding more local anesthetic during the procedure.

Another potential complication is related to poor eyebrow density. This is most likely because of lower than expected percentage of hair regrowth. Despite the best efforts to keep the grafts moist, as well as the atraumatic placement of the grafts, in certain cases 20% to 25% of the hair may fail to regrow. To minimize poor regrowth rates, the grafts are kept "chubby" with a small cuff of surrounding protective fat, and the most experienced assistants perform the insertion of the grafts. Patients are advised that this is not necessarily a complication, but rather something that simply sometimes occur, and thus a second smaller procedure can be performed after 10 months or more to achieve greater density.

Lastly, poor hair growth angulation can occur in the occasional case despite the best efforts in acute recipient site angulation and hair placement. This is likely because of the effects of healing and subtle wound contracture. It is most commonly seen in patients with straight hair, in whom the harvesting of the natural curl to assure flat growth of hairs is difficult. To best prevent this, an acute angle is taken with the skin when making recipient sites and rotating the hair on insertion, so that the natural curl of the hair is aimed downward. It is also best not to trim the hair in the donor area—if by strip method—to better visualize the hair curl.

Postprocedure Care

Patients are instructed to keep the eyebrows dry for the first 5 days. If strip harvesting was performed, sutures are removed approximately 10 days postoperatively, or the dissolvable sutures are expected to be gone by 4 weeks. Antibiotics and pain medications are given for the first several days. Patients are allowed to use makeup in the eyebrow area after all the crusts have fallen out at typically 5 days.

Eyebrows will start to regrow 4 to 6 months after transplant and will continue to fill in for a full year, gradually increasing in density. A variety of products can be used to train any misdirected hairs. The hair must be trimmed to the patient's desired length. If a patient so desires, second smaller procedures to increase density are performed 10 months or later.

REFERENCES

1. Rassman WR, Berstein RM, McClellan R, et al. Follicular unit extraction: minimally invasive surgery for hair transplantation. Dermatol Surg 2002;28:720–8.
2. Harris J. Conventional FUE in hair transplantation. In: Unger W, Shapiro R, Unger R, editors. Hair transplantation. 5th edition. New York: Thieme; 2001. p. 291–6.
3. Donor area harvesting. In: Unger W, Shapiro R, Unger R, et al, editors. Hair transplantation. 5th edition. New York: Thieme; 2011. p. 247–90.
4. Gandelman M, Epstein JS. Reconstruction of the sideburn, moustache, and beard. Facial Plast Surg Clin North Am 2004;12:253–61.
5. Epstein JS. Hair restoration to eyebrows, beard, sideburns, and eyelashes. Facial Plast Surg Clin North Am 2013;21:457–67.
6. Tosti A, Piraccini BM. Diagnosis and treatment of hair disorders: an evidence based atlas. New York: Informa Healthcare; 2005.

The Modified Upper Lip Lift

Advanced Approach with Deep-Plane Release and Secure Suspension: 823-Patient Series

Benjamin Talei, MD

KEYWORDS

- Modified upper lip lift • Philtrum • Reduction • Shortening • Augmentation

KEY POINTS

- Deep-plane release of the SMAS tissue in the upper lip permits a tension-free suspension to the ligaments at the nasal base.
- Preoperative incision and vector markings provide a map for proper skin redistribution.
- Suspension suturing of the deep lip tissue allows proper, tension-free, healing in a highly dynamic region.
- Immaculate closure is of utmost importance at the nasal base.
- Techniques crossing the nasal sill should be avoided.

INTRODUCTION
The Evolution of Lip Lifting

The upper lip lift has been performed for over 4 decades.[1] The modified upper lip lift takes established principles used elsewhere in facial surgery and applies them to upper lip rejuvenation to obtain superior results. Traditional lip lift techniques have been criticized and often avoided out of the fear of scarring. To avoid problems that can be encountered at the nasal base, surgeons have become increasingly creative with incision design, trying to maximize results and decrease complications. Unfortunately, few of these techniques have provided esthetically natural and reproducible results.

The bullhorn subnasal lip lift was one of the first acceptable techniques, as described in 1971 by Cardoso and Sperli.[1] Several renditions followed with the goal of reducing incision length, limiting scarring and enhancing the amount of lifting.[2–6] Unfortunately, most of these techniques have a tendency toward nasal base effacement and scarring that is difficult to repair according to the author's clinical experience (**Figs. 1–4**).

Our technique is based on the classic bullhorn incision with modifications that have made a significant improvement in results and consistency. Rather than focus on changes in incision design, the key to our procedure is a deeper and more extensive release of the upper lip and more definitive suspension. The modified upper lip lift is a centrally vectored deep-plane advancement flap focused on releasing tension in the skin and uniformly redistributing the skin once tethering is released. The preoperative radial vector markings designed and depicted by the author are essential to optimizing outcomes. We performed 823 upper lip lifts over the 4-year period from 01/01/2015 until

Disclosure Statement: The author has nothing to disclose.
Facial Plastic & Reconstructive Surgery, Beverly Hills Center for Plastic & Laser Surgery, 465 North Roxbury Drive, Suite 750, Beverly Hills, CA 90210, USA
E-mail address: drtalei@beverlyhillscenter.com

Facial Plast Surg Clin N Am 27 (2019) 385–398
https://doi.org/10.1016/j.fsc.2019.04.004
1064-7406/19/© 2019 Elsevier Inc. All rights reserved.

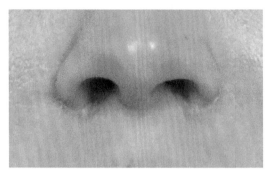

Fig. 1. Atrophic scarring with nasal effacement following "Italian Lip Lift."

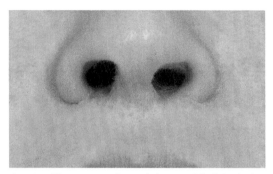

Fig. 3. Effacement of nasal base with labial skin pulled into the nose with loss of sill volume.

the date of this article 10/31/2018. Review of our results reveals consistent outcomes with few complications when using our technique for the modified upper lip lift.

PATIENT SELECTION

The modifications made to the bullhorn subnasal lip lift technique have allowed a significantly wider application of this procedure. Previously reserved primarily for elderly patients with light skin, this procedure can now be used on patients of a wide variety of ages, skin types, genders, and ethnicities. This procedure can also be used for patients with already adequate tooth show who wish to improve upper lip height, character, and volume. Even the most conservative upper lip lift can change the slope and vector of the vermillion and make the lip more receptive to filler augmentation (**Figs. 5–7**).

The most common presentations and complaints in the author's practice are shown in **Box 1**.

Patients often present with excess lip length and drooping, complaining of looking tired and aged. An elongated upper lip can lengthen the appearance of the entire midface. Lack of tooth show exaggerates the aged appearance and can

dramatically diminish sensuality. As the lip lengthens, it also tends to display diminished function while losing character and definition of the Cupid's bow (**Figs. 8–10**).

In recent years, there has been an emergence of patients suffering the negative effects of fillers. Permanent fillers such as silicone, fat, and other polymers such as polymethylmethacrylate (PMMA) may cause perpetual damage to the upper lip because of expansion, thickening, and effacement. They may also dramatically inhibit lip function through muscular infiltration and/or edema. The upper lip lift cannot restore the lip to a normal state, but it can re-elevate the lip to a higher position with improved eversion and improve overall appearance (**Figs. 11 and 12**).

Temporary injectables such as hyaluronic acid (HLA) dermal fillers may have negative short-term outcomes, as well as permanent sequelae. The most notorious of these fillers to have a problem is Juvderm XC. Due to it being hydrophilic from its high HLA concentration (24 mg/mL) and migratory in nature, it accounts for most problems seen with HLA products in my practice. The tissue integration and migration of this product can cause a spreading out of the filler in the subcutaneous

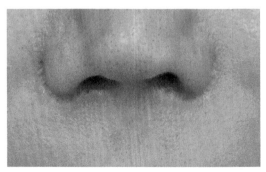

Fig. 2. Atrophic scarring with striations after vertical lifting with extended lateral incisions.

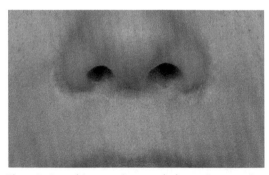

Fig. 4. Atrophic scarring and hypopigmentation following upper lip lift performed with high tension closure.

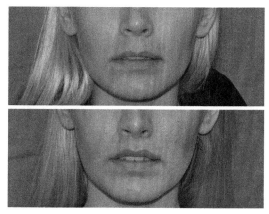

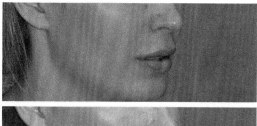

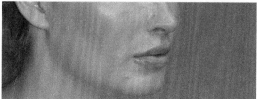

Fig. 5. Conservative excision on a patient with adequate tooth show improving lip accents.

Fig. 7. Conservative excision improving lip accent and appearance.

tissue of the lip, beyond the vermillion border where it was injected. The author has witnessed the persistence of Juvederm in reactive regions for over 8 years. Given the issues witnessed following injections of Juvederm XC, PMMA, silicone, and other polymers, the author has advised against their use in the lips. Fat injections in the lip may have similar consequences, and fat grafting should not be done without prejudice. These migratory, hydrophilic, and inflammatory fillers are most notably found within the 10-mm segment above the vermillion border months to years following injection (**Figs. 13–16**). They are quite noticeable on most patients, presenting with a bulge, whitish discoloration, simian upper lip convexity, and limitation in smile. Dissolving HLA filler above the vermillion border is easy to do and should be done before pursuing surgical intervention to increase precision and decrease postoperative inflammation.

Another presenting complaint is drooping or lengthening of the upper lip following surgical

procedures such as rhinoplasty or orthognathic surgery. Rhinoplasty can have a clear and direct effect on the position of the upper lip. Maneuvers that deproject the nasal tip, such as transfixion incisions or dissection around the nasal base, can cause the lip to lower immediately or shortly after surgery. This can be prevented, reversed, or improved using a variety of resuspension techniques such as the "tongue-in-groove" maneuver, suspension to the nasal spine, or by performing an upper lip lift.

Another common presenting patient issue is asymmetry of the upper lip. Complaints typically include height disparities between Cupid's bow peaks, differences with smiling, and position of the oral commissures. Mild asymmetries at the Cupid's bow and along the adjacent vermillion may be improved in some cases, but more lateral or more significant asymmetries are typically beyond the scope of an upper lip lift (see **Fig. 16**). Most lateral lip asymmetries are a consequence of facial asymmetries, which are not amenable to improvement from a procedure done at the base of the nose.

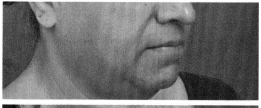

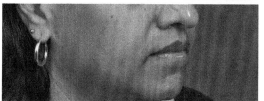

Fig. 6. Lip eversion following modified upper lip lift providing improved vermillion vectoring and display.

Box 1
Common complaints

1. Chronically long or heavy upper lip
2. Poor tooth show/dental hooding
3. Over-filled lips/poor filler results
4. Filler complications
5. Postsurgical drooping (rhinoplasty/orthognathic)
6. Poorly defined or thin upper lip
7. Asymmetry
8. Buried or drooping corners of the mouth
9. Upper lip incompetence

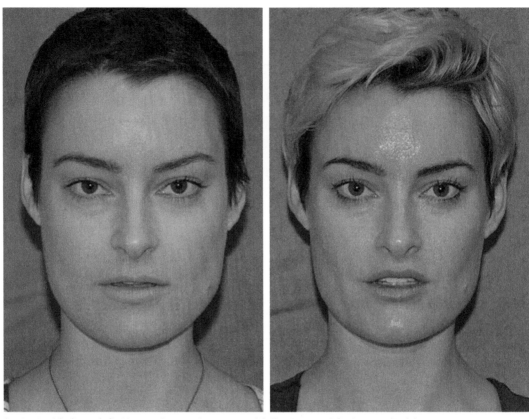

Fig. 8. Cupid's bow definition and sensuality restored following modified upper lip lift.

SURGICAL TECHNIQUE
Dental and Facial Analysis

The threshold for patient candidacy is significantly lower when using the modified upper lip lift technique. The exceptions are patients in whom a lip lift would create imbalance or an exaggerated appearance. A familiarity with minimum and maximum excision amounts, as well as the necessary minimum height of lip to be left in situ is of great importance. However, the true art of lip lifting

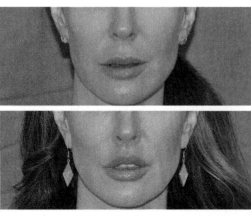

Fig. 9. Youth and tooth show restored following modified upper lip lift.

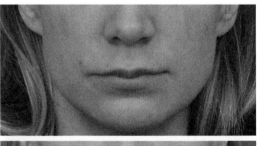

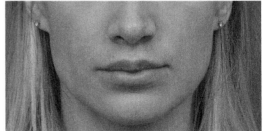

Fig. 10. Cupid's bow definition tightened following modified upper lip lift.

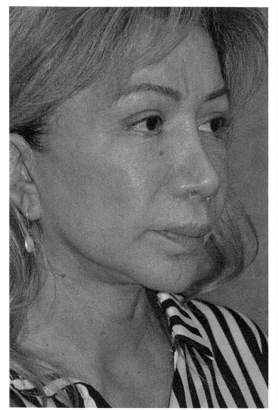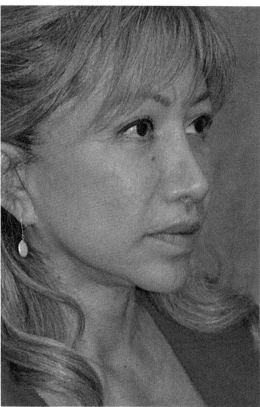

Fig. 11. Modified upper lip lift combined with nasal base suspension and mucosal excision to improve silicone-caused deformities.

comes from a thorough facial analysis and an ability to "eyeball" what would look good.

Overall facial balance must be considered, comparing soft tissue proportions, as well as dental or skeletal predominance. A primary goal of the lip lift for most patients and practitioners is to increase the incisive tooth show. There is a tipping point that must be respected for each patient, where the sensuality and youthfulness gained from increased tooth show transitions to a toothy or skeletonized appearance with excessive excision. There are no measurements or strict

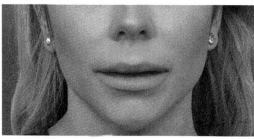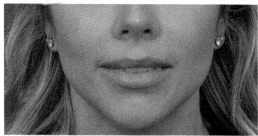

Fig. 13. Front view. Top photo demonstrating simian appearance and heaviness from Juvederm. Bottom photo after dissolver and lip lift.

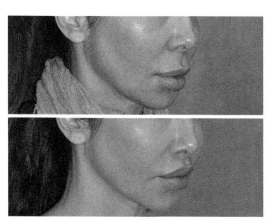

Fig. 12. Upper lip weighing down from fillers now resuspended following modified upper lip lift.

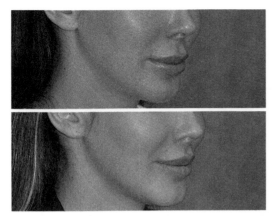

Fig. 14. Corner view. Top photo demonstrating simian appearance and heaviness from Juvederm. Bottom photo after dissolver and lip lift.

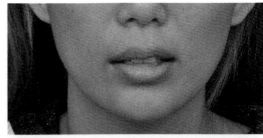

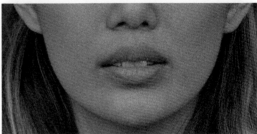

Fig. 16. Mild asymmetries improved with an asymmetric lip lift. Normal healing in Asian skin types.

guidelines that would indicate this level or point. A 3-mm tooth show on a patient with beautiful teeth and normal projection may be lovely, whereas the same amount of tooth show on a patient with a strong dental overjet (type II malocclusion), malocclusion, a gaunt facial appearance, or unappealing dentition may be excessive. Surprisingly, "gummy smiles" are rarely affected or exaggerated with the modified upper lip lift, likely because this technique has the ability to decrease the exertion or strain on the upper lip with smiling (**Fig. 17**).

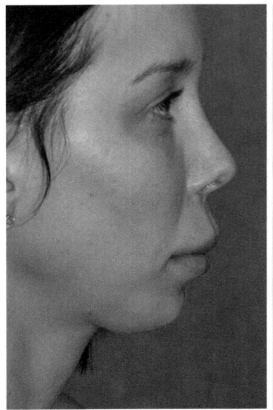

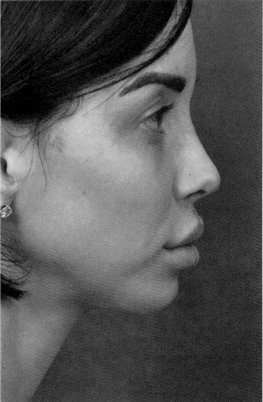

Fig. 15. Lateral view. Top photo demonstrating simian appearance, projection, and heaviness from Juvederm. Bottom photo after dissolver and lip lift.

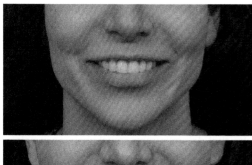

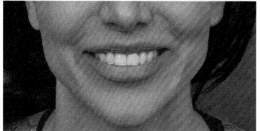

Fig. 17. A more relaxed smile noted in the bottom photo after modified upper lip lift.

Excessive tooth show, maxillary-mandibular imbalance, or unappealing dentition should not preclude one from performing a lip lift. Either a conservative lip lift may be performed, in the 3- to 5-mm range of excision, or the patient may first be referred to a cosmetic dentist, orthognathic surgeon, or orthodontist.

Relative soft tissue balance is also important. We learn to begin by analyzing the horizontal fifth's and the vertical thirds of the face, but there are many variables affecting what we perceive as a pleasant harmony of the face. The proportions we see on patients with thick skin or a full-round face may be drastically different than that of a patient with a thin or delicate face. Rather than measure the proportions directly, the author recommends looking at the face as a whole and simply envisioning the changes to be made. The overall intent is to make the lip fit appropriately in relation to its surrounding structures, primarily the nose, cheeks, and chin. For example, a wide nasal base with fatty ala and flaring will not tolerate the appearance of a foreshortened upper lip.

Surgical Marking

The excision outline and radial reference markings designed by the author are the most crucial part of this procedure. The markings are based on the classic "bullhorn" lip lift. The excision and closure should be treated as a centrally vectored advancement flap. The markings are made in a step-wise and logical fashion to aid in the decision of the proper amount of upper lip excision and to make the design as symmetric possible.

1. The first step is to mark the upper incision (**Fig. 18**). This mark goes across the entire nasal base in the natural alar-facial and alar-labial crease. The lateral extent of this is where the alar-facial crease tapers and ends caudally toward the alar groove. The incision should not go past the superior or lateral extent of the well-demarcated crease, which may end on the inferior or lateral part of the ala. Extending an incision beyond this point may cause distortion and scarring of the crease or even create a pleat from the cheek to the nose and efface the natural upper lateral extent of the upper lip esthetic unit. The incision continues under the nose, making sure not to invade the nasal sill. In hypotrophic nasal sills, a healthy amount of tissue must deliberately be left in situ. Progressing centrally, the marking will reach a peak either at the superior extent of the philtral column or at the divergence of the medial crural footplate around the nasal spine. It is important to note that the line of the philtral column and this peak do not always align. Moving further centrally, the 2 paramedian peaks then transition into a dip at the junction of the lip to the base of the columella. This crease may be low and buried or high at the base of a rotated columella.

2. Two reference markings are made on each side, extending radially from the internal sill and the external rim. The height of excision is then demarcated (**Fig. 19**). The best starting point on most patients is on a horizontal crease or line that the author deems a "line of declaration." Most patients with an elongated lip have 1 or 2 horizontal creases that form in lines of tension during strained smiling. If this is not present, the next step would be to find an area of transition or inflexion on the upper lip following the base of the columella inferiorly. Most lips

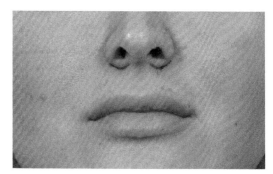

Fig. 18. The first step in marking is to find the natural crease between the nose and lip. The lateral-most extent should be at the transition zone between a well-defined and blunted crease. Medially the peak occurs where the medial crural footplate diverges.

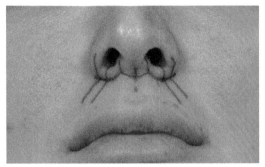

Fig. 19. Radial reference markings are made to aid even distribution and advancement of flaps from the internal sill following the curve of the lip outward as well as from the alar rim margin. The 2 paramedian peaks are marked along with the center of the columella. The ideal height is marked.

look maximally appealing if they begin with a vertical slope, transitioning anteriorly toward the vermillion like a ski ramp (**Figs. 20** and **21**). Once this point is chosen, the surgeon must determine the ideal location for the best looking lip with an incision that would yield the ideal excision for perfect tooth show. As a security measure, mark the minimum amount of remaining lip. For most patients, this would be around 11 mm as measured from the Cupid's bow peak superiorly while the lip is on stretch. Leaving less than 10 mm of residual upper lip height is not recommended.

The amount of expected tooth show gained from each excisional height is demonstrated in

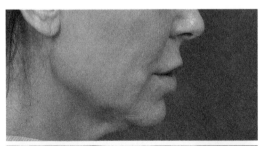

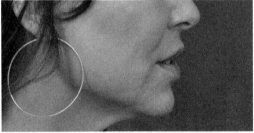

Fig. 20. The upper lip looks most pleasant with an immediate transition from vertical to sloped.

Table 1. These measurements should only serve as guidelines. The amount to be excised typically ranges between 4 and 11 mm, with most standard excisions ranging between 5 and 7 mm. Excisions aiming for notable tooth show are typically between 7 and 9 mm. An excision of over 11 mm is not advised, because this dramatically increases healing time and makes redistribution of skin difficult for the average patient. There are many variables that determine the actual changes in height including skin thickness, skin laxity, muscle function, and nasal base laxity. The lift obtained on patients with thinner upper lips tends to be more exaggerated than on those patients with thick or hyperelastic lips (see **Table 1**).

Once the excision height is marked, a caliper is used to measure the distance with the lip on stretch. The lower incision marking is then made using a caliper uniformly and in parallel to the upper incision, until the first of the lateral radial markings is encountered (**Fig. 22**). At this point, the dots are connected between the internal rim reference marking and the peak of the lateral upper incision. If there is a minor Cupid's bow asymmetry, this can be corrected at this stage, with an asymmetric excision. Lateral asymmetries cannot be corrected with a surgery centered at the base of the nose.

Once all the dots are connected, the remaining reference markings are drawn, totaling 9 lines. A vertical marking is placed on each incision peak and 1 in the center. Intermediate markings are then made between the peak marking and the internal rim marking (**Fig. 23**). These points serve as closure points for the deep suspension sutures as well as even centralized redistribution markings for the advancement of the lower flap.

Excision

The procedure is performed using local anesthesia and with the surgeon at the head of the bed. The lower incision is made first, with a 15 blade scalpel perpendicular to skin, extending to the junction of the fat and the muscle. The upper incision is then made parallel to the lower incision (**Fig. 24**). The skin and subcutaneous flap is then excised in a plane over the orbicularis, leaving a thin glossy layer of fat intact. This glossy layer is where most of the vasculature lays deep to the superficial muscular aponeurotic system (SMAS). The larger-caliber vessels in the field are the inferior alar arteries, which are buried under the ala and alar sill, running parallel to them (**Fig. 25**).

Dissection

Once the excision is performed, the labial flap is then elevated in a deep sub-SMAS plane. This

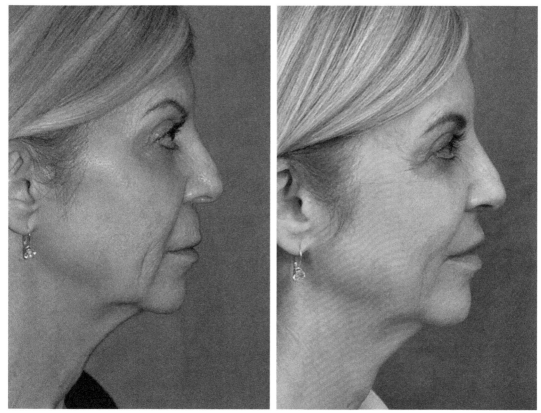

Fig. 21. The upper lip convexity in the before photo causes an aged, simian appearance.

dissection releases the labial SMAS from the underlying orbicularis oris. The extent of this dissection is at the discretion of the surgeon, as more extensive dissection may mitigate tension but also causes a dramatic increase in postoperative swelling. Taller excisions typically require a greater degree of release, as do patients who require release and rolling of the lateral vermillion to avoid a subsequent corner lift. The average patient will require release in the deep plane half-way down the central philtrum. Full central dissection is avoided because of possible effacement of the Cupid's bow (**Figs. 26** and **27**). Laterally, the dissection is carried as far out as necessary to

obtain a palpable release of the labial flap that would allow a minimal tension closure. For most patients the dissection approaches or extends to the vermillion anywhere lateral to the philtral columns and stops just before the nasolabial fold. Care must be taken to stay in a directly sub-SMAS plane to avoid excessive bleeding or damage to any of the labial elevator complex. Careful hemostasis must be achieved, preferably with a bipolar cautery (**Fig. 28**). Although a hematoma is not typically a risk in classic lip lifts, it is a consideration with a modified upper lip lift given the extensive dissection and dead space created.

Suspension and Closure

The mistake made by most practitioners is performing a simple dermal closure. As we have learned from endoscopic brow lifting and advanced forms of face lifting, the best lift is achieved by performing adequate release of tethering and then by suspension of dense tissue upward to a fixed location. When this is performed in the upper lip, the released skin/SMAS flap is then able to roll over and redistribute tension above the contracted orbicularis.

Table 1
Estimated lift based on excision height—variable

Excision (mm)	3	4	5	6	7	8	9	10	11
Tooth show (mm)	0	0–1	1–2	2–3	2–4	3–5	4–6	5–7	6–8

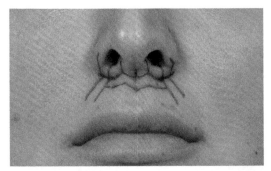

Fig. 22. Castro-Viejo angles caliper is used to mark the height of excision with the lip on stretch. Equal heights are marked between the internal sill reference markings.

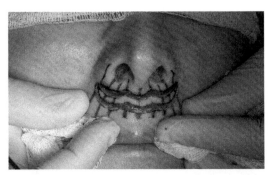

Fig. 24. Perpendicular incisions are made through the skin, fat, and SMAS to the level of the orbicularis layer. Upper and lower incisions are made in parallel to aide in proper approximation.

The dermis at the base of the nose is not firmly attached. The periosteum or overlying pyriform ligament are the only firm structures that can provide a strong base for suspension. Suturing to the periostium produces an over exaggerated tacking of the labial flap. The pyriform ligament is a dense network of fibrous tissue overlying the periosteum that spans the pyriform aperture and is perfect for engagement of suspensory sutures.[7]

A 5-0 PDS suture on a P-3 needle is used at each of the central 7 reference markings. The needle is passed into the junction of the nasal and oral musculature and then carried deep to grab the pyriform ligament but not the periosteum. The needle exits deep to the alar dermis with care not to incorporate the dermis (**Fig. 29**). The needle is then passed inferiorly through the SMAS on the underside of the labial flap (**Fig. 30**). The SMAS of the upper lip is a discrete tissue layer with substantial strength that is located just deep to the reticular dermis.[8,9]

Suturing to the SMAS instead of the dermis allows the skin to approximate without tension or

dimpling. This provides a major advantage by pushing the dermal edges together. The incision is closed sequentially from central to lateral (**Fig. 31**). Once the knots are tied, the skin edges should be closely approximated. At the lateralmost reference marking, a 4-0 Vicryl on a PS-2 needle is passed from inside the pyriform coming out radially to grab the SMAS, and then returned back into the nose to complete a mattress suture (**Fig. 32**). The inferior alar artery should be identified and avoided, if possible. The skin is then reapproximated with a plethora of vertical mattress and interrupted 6-0 nylon sutures, with the end point being resolution of any step-offs from the lower to upper skin flaps (**Figs. 33** and **34**). This area is unforgiving and meticulous suturing technique is required.

POSTOPERATIVE COURSE
Postoperative Care

The incisions must be kept moist with ointment at all times in the first several weeks. Patients are given a surgical mask to so they do not feel self-

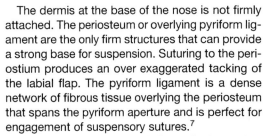

Fig. 23. The remainder of the inferior marking is made by tapering from the internal sill markings upward. The corresponding reference markings are made, as well as 2 intermediate reference markings to total 9 markings.

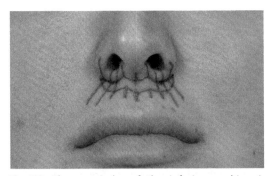

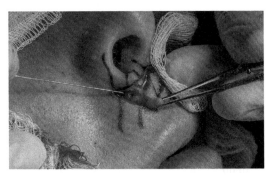

Fig. 25. The marked skin, fat, and SMAS are excised leaving a thin, glossy fat layer intact to avoid damage of vessels and the inferior alar artery marked in the photo.

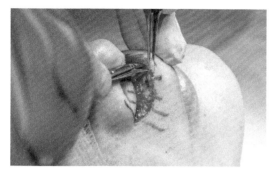

Fig. 26. Deep-plane/sub-SMAS elevation is performed directly over the muscle layer.

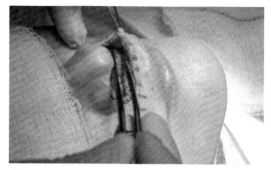

Fig. 28. Hemostasis is obtained using bipolar electro-cautery to minimize risk of hematoma.

conscious. Sutures are typically removed partially at day 3 and completely at day 5 (**Fig. 35**). Taping is neither affective nor necessary. Patients are forewarned that swelling may appear extreme and that the appearance of the lip typically takes 3 months to return to normal. Relative to others, this technique produces significantly more swelling in this area because of the disruption of bilateral lymphatic drainage pathways as well as muscle trauma causing a postoperative myositis. The stiffness and swelling in the first 3 months may benefit incisional healing by limiting movement at the incision line. Patients are seen at 3-week intervals for reassurance and potential injection of 5-fluorouracil 50mg/cc into a firm orbicularis patch. The nasal base is also quite responsive to fractionated CO_2 laser, should that be required. Most patients receive this routinely at 60 and 120 days at a low setting.

Potential Sequelae

The most commonly encountered sequelae of an upper lip lift are scarring and widening of the nasal base. For this reason, most practitioners who perform the lip lift procedure do so on elderly patients with light skin. Issues can arise with any

technique. However, when using the bullhorn incision, even if unsightly scarring occurs, it can most often be easily and significantly improved with scar modulation therapies. Off-label use of 5-fluorouracil 50mg/cc can help flatten hypertrophic incisions. CO_2 laser can improve hypertrophic, atrophic, and other types of scarring.

Alternative techniques that involve more complex types of incisions, such as the philtral stretching variations of the upper lip lift, L-shaped philtrum lift, extended incision lip lift, Greenwald incision, double duck suspension, and the Italian technique, may result in greater amounts of scarring and changes to the nasal base that are difficult to reverse. Atrophic scarring is quite common, as well as skeletonization or effacement of the nasal base. Incisions extending into the nasal sill inherently cut away healthy mass and volume at the nasal base while advancing the skin of the lip inside the nose where it does not naturally reside.

Distortion or effacement of the nasal base can occur with untoward tension on compliant portions of the nasal base. When tension is combined with excision of portions of nasal sill, the distortion can become more prominent. If the central lip is lifted or excised more than the lateral portions,

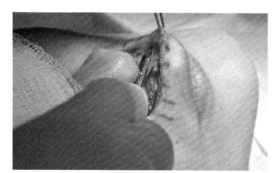

Fig. 27. Sub-SMAS dissection is continued half-way down the central philtrum. Lateral dissection is typically carried to the same level or greater.

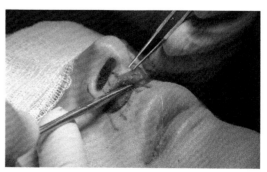

Fig. 29. 5-0 PDS suture enters between the nasal and labial muscle layers, passes deep grabbing the pyriform ligament, and exits just deep to the dermis.

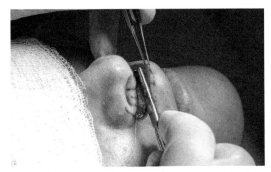

Fig. 30. The 5-0 PDS is passed deep to the dermis to grab the SMAS layer only.

this can also produce an unnatural and disproportionate postoperative appearance to the lip that further exaggerates a suboptimal outcome. Central lip lifts are rarely indicated and most commonly produce an exaggerated upturn of the central lip. This often results in relative worsening of the appearance of lateral lip hooding. It is important to remember that there are limits to what a procedure at the nasal base can achieve. The intent to change the character of the lip significantly should be avoided.

Avoiding Sequelae

The first way to assure a superior result is proper incision design, following the principles of the bullhorn lip lift. This means avoiding cutting into and damaging the nasal sill by carrying incisions inside the nose. Most techniques that involve hidden incisions inherently require that healthy sill skin is excised and replaced with skin from the lip. Labial skin does not naturally occur within the nasal sill and it should not be placed there during a strictly cosmetic procedure. Once the sill is removed and scarring occurs, the sill cannot be replaced and the atrophic skin that replaces it is quite difficult to repair.

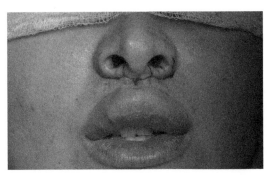

Fig. 32. The 7 central reference markings are closed with the deep layer of 5-0 PDS sutures. The 2 most lateral markings are closed using a 4-0 Vicryl entering from the inside of the nose, passing externally between the orbicularis muscle and nasal ala to grab the SMAS layer then exit through the nose by passing through the nasolabial junction.

Problematic healing also seems to arise from inadequate incision length and insufficient deep tissue release. Making smaller incisions, whether single in the center or bilateral incisions under the nasal sills, tend to increase complications as well. Smaller incisions may limit the proper release of tension and redistribution of skin, while also presenting the potential for disproportionate lifting. This means that, although incisions are limited, there may be higher tension placed on each incision point, resulting in poor healing. Uniform redistribution avoids irregularities and skin bunching by spreading the tension evenly along the length of the entire incision. The perioral region is extremely dynamic, and all possible efforts to relieve tension at the incision should be performed. Proper release of the deep structures to reduce closure tension, coupled with adequate deep suturing, followed by intricate superficial suturing, will enhance results. The practitioner should be aware that the nasal base is an unforgiving area with regard to

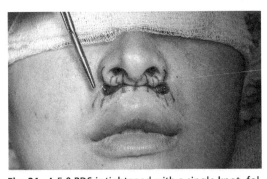

Fig. 31. A 5-0 PDS is tightened with a single knot, followed by a slip knot, then a locking knot.

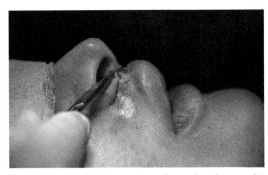

Fig. 33. Superficial closure is performed with a combination of 6-0 nylon vertical mattress and interrupted sutures.

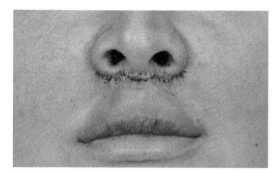

Fig. 34. Closure using enough sutures to avoid any step-offs or irregularities.

irregularities and scarring. Although it may not seem so, longer incisions tend to heal better than shorter ones.

Some lip lifting techniques rely on muscle suspension, excision, or plication to relieve tension on the skin.[6,10] This ideology may theoretically be supported by muscle-tightening procedures performed during facelift surgery; however, mimetic muscles are not routinely suspended during rhytidectomy. Rather, the SMAS-platysma complex is tightened, which carries no mimetic function. A dense SMAS fascia definitively exists in the upper lip just deep to the dermis and superficial to the orbicularis oris muscle. The SMAS-skin flap may be released and used for lifting similar to deep-plane lifting in the face. The orbicularis oris is a mimetic muscle that is extremely dynamic and sensitive to trauma. From the author's experience, muscle binding has a higher probability of causing fibrosis at the plicated region and may actually have a tendency to pull the nasal base in a downward direction. Still, muscle plication or imbrication may serve a purpose in some patients during various lip lifting procedures including the modified upper lip lift. When binding is performed during this procedure, it is typically limited to the uppermost 2 mm of the orbicularis muscle. The

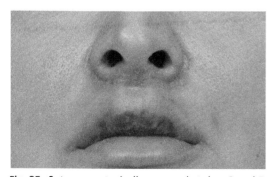

Fig. 35. Sutures are typically removed at days 3 and 5. This photos was taken 5 days postoperatively.

upper orbicularis is taken and suspended to the pyriform ligament using 5-0 PDS sutures to limit potential damage to the muscle and nasal base. Experienced practitioners may use muscle-binding techniques routinely with high success rates, but amount of muscle trauma in the hands of the novice surgeon should be limited.

Direct vermillion excisions tend to cause a blurring of the vermillion and a visible scar with a potentially unnatural appearance that almost always requires lip liner camouflage. Once the vermillion is distorted, it cannot be recreated. In the author's opinion, the only indication for an incision at the vermillion border is the rare patient who requires a corner of the mouth lift.[11] Corner lift incisions are limited and seldom cause issues; however, we perform them rarely because the modified upper lip lift has the ability to treat this region on most patients.

Complications

A chart review of 823 consecutive lip lifts from January 2015 to October 2018 in the author's private practice was performed. Histories were reviewed for any complications seen past the 3-month mark. Of note, there were no patients demonstrating any limitation in movement or smile. Five patients required revision to obtain further lifting or further lifting and symmetry. Two patients developed dermal atrophy and telangiectasias following injection with triamcinolone. Because of this, the author no longer injects triamcinolone postoperatively in these patients. Two patients complained of vague changes in character of the nostrils, which were difficult to depict in photos. Two patients experienced minor hematomas, which were limited by tamponade. Two patients had prolonged edema extending to the 4-month mark, which then resolved. Both of these patients had previous silicone injections and an 11-mm excision. Ten patients developed a rash from antibiotic ointment. Two patients presented with a 1-mm rim of eschar/epidermolysis of unknown cause around the lateral nostril base that healed without incidence. Although many patients received scar modulation with injections of 5-fluorouracil 50mg/cc and/or CO_2 laser treatments on the incisions, none were bothered by their incisions. There were no patients found to have increasing asymmetry. There were no incidents of infection.

Forty-five patients had a simultaneous lip lift with rhinoplasty with no adverse sequelae. Alarplasty was performed at a separate time on all but 2 patients to avoid lateral scarring. Sixty-two patients had simultaneous lip lift with rhytidectomy with no adverse sequelae. Sixty-eight patients had simultaneous mucosal lip reductions mostly to reduce polymer-related abnormalities. Fifteen received simultaneous dermis or SMAS grafts to augment lip volume and there were no adverse effects. One patient requested a subsequent corner lift. The remainder of the patients seeking corner lifting before surgery received an adequate degree from the modified upper lip lift.

SUMMARY

A variety of lip lift techniques have been created over time with the intent of diminishing scarring and poor outcomes. A great deal of energy has been misdirected toward compensatory measures such as changes in incision design rather than simply improving the manner in which the lip is lifted. The modified upper lip lift is a sub-SMAS release and suspension technique that simplifies procedural steps and minimizes risks of adverse outcomes. Furthermore, it permits a wider application of an often-needed technique to all ages, ethnicities, genders, and skin types. We have learned a great deal from other facial cosmetic surgeries, such as brow lifts, upper blepharoplasty, and deep-plane rhytidectomy. As guided by the evolution of upper blepharoplasty, muscle preservation is essential for maintaining proper function and volume. Face-lifting techniques have demonstrated a much greater efficacy when tension is adequately released then resuspended to a firm or fixed structure, such as is seen with deep-plane facelifts.

The upper lip lift has the ability to produce a high yield change on the face with a single, small procedure. It can produce a younger and more sensual appearance by shortening the perceived height of the midface, as well as by increasing tooth show and oral visibility. The nasolabial fold in most patients appears softer and shortened as well. This easily reproducible technique has repeatedly demonstrated consistent outcomes with an exceedingly low complication rate. The need for such a procedure is under-recognized in patients of all ages. The modified upper lip lift is a safe, consistent, reproducible, and widely applicable technique for any gender, ethnicity, and skin type.

REFERENCES

1. Cardoso AD, Sperli AE. Rhytidoplasty of the upper lip. Transactions of the fifth international congress of plastic and reconstructive surgery. Sydney (Australia): Butterworth-Heinemann; 1971. p. 1127–9.
2. Gonzalez-Ulloa M. The aging upper lip. Ann Plast Surg 1979;2(4):299–303.
3. Austin HW. The lip lift. Plast Reconstr Surg 1986; 77(6):990–4.
4. Greenwald AE. The lip lift. Plast Reconstr Surg 1987; 79(1):147.
5. Cardim VL, dos Santos Silva A, De Faria Valle R, et al. "Double duck" nasolabial lifting. Rev Bras Cir Plást 2011;26:466–71.
6. Santachè P, Bonarrigo C. Lifting of the upper lip: personal technique. Plast Reconstr Surg 2004;113: 1828–35.
7. Rohrich RJ, Hoxworth RE, Thornton JF, et al. The pyriform ligament. Plast Reconstr Surg 2008;121(1): 277–81.
8. Sandulescu T, Spilker L, Rauscher D, et al. Morphological analysis and three-dimensional reconstruction of the SMAS surrounding the nasolabial fold. Ann Anat 2018;217:111–7.
9. Ghassemi A, Prescher A, Riediger D, et al. Anatomy of the SMAS revisited. Aesthetic Plast Surg 2003; 27(4):258–64.
10. Pan BL. Upper lip lift with a "T"-shaped resection of the orbicularis oris muscle for Asian perioral rejuvenation: a report of 84 patients. J Plast Reconstr Aesthet Surg 2017;70(3):392–400.
11. Weston GW, Poindexter BD, Sigal RK, et al. Lifting lips: 28 years of experience using the direct excision approach to rejuvenating the aging mouth. Aesthet Surg J 2009;29(2):83–6.

The Critical Role of Nutrition in Facial Plastic Surgery

Frédérick Laliberté, MD[a], Ilan Bloom, BEng, MES[b,1],
Ashlin J. Alexander, MD, FRCSC[c,*]

KEYWORDS

- Surgical nutrition • Healing • Surgery • Facial plastic surgery • Wound healing

KEY POINTS

- Malnutrition has been shown to be a modifiable risk factor for increased morbidity and mortality in patients undergoing surgery.
- Incorporating nutritional interventions in the perioperative care of cosmetic surgery patients may help correct subclinical dietary deficiencies, accelerate recovery, and improve surgical outcomes.
- Key nutrients include vitamin A, vitamin C, zinc, bromelain, arnica montana, arginine, glutamine, hydrolyzed collagen, vitamin B complex, and protein.

INTRODUCTION

Recent research has led to a greater appreciation of the critical impact of nutrition on health and disease. Through a series of crucial discoveries in the nineteenth century, scientists compiled an extensive list of nutrients necessary for normal physiologic function. These nutrients, referred to as "essential nutrients," are not synthesized by the human body and thus must be obtained from dietary sources.[1] In the present day, nutrition plays a fundamental role in modern medicine, with dietary modifications forming the basis of how we treat and prevent cardiovascular, endocrine, inflammatory, and oncologic diseases.

The same is true in the surgical field, as clinical nutrition is now considered an important determinant of surgical outcome. Moreover, nutrition can be harnessed to optimize healing and provide superior results from surgery. The goal of this article is to review the role of nutrition in today's surgical patient, and, more specifically, in the realm of facial plastic and reconstructive surgery.

RISK OF MALNUTRITION

There is an abundance of literature demonstrating the benefits of adequate nutrition in hospitalized patients. A prospective study performed by Schneider and colleagues[2] in nonselected hospital inpatients demonstrated that malnutrition was an independent risk factor for the development of nosocomial infections (odds ratio [OR] 4.98; 95% confidence interval [CI] 4.0–6.40). The importance of nutrition in surgery has also been extensively studied, particularly in the general surgery population. Kuzu and colleagues[3] performed

Disclosure Statement: Dr A.J. Alexander is on the Advisory Board for Nutrition for Healing LLC, the company which produces MEND Cosmetic, as well as a shareholder in Nutrition for Healing LLC. Drs I. Bloom and Laliberte have nothing to disclose.
[a] Division of Facial Plastic and Reconstructive Surgery, Department of Otolaryngology-Head & Neck Surgery, University of Toronto, 190 Elizabeth Street, Room 3S438, RFE Building, Toronto, Ontario M5G 2C4, Canada;
[b] Douglas Hospital Research Center, McGill University; [c] Division of Facial Plastic and Reconstructive Surgery, Department of Otolaryngology-Head & Neck Surgery, University of Toronto, Toronto, Ontario, Canada
[1] Present address: 6875 Boulevard Lasalle, Montréal, Québec H4H 1R3, Canada.
* Corresponding author. 251 Davenport Road, Toronto, Ontario, M5R1J9, Canada.
E-mail address: ASHLIN@ASHLINALEXANDER.COM

Facial Plast Surg Clin N Am 27 (2019) 399–404
https://doi.org/10.1016/j.fsc.2019.04.005
1064-7406/19/© 2019 Elsevier Inc. All rights reserved.

a prospective trial of 460 patients undergoing major elective surgery. They demonstrated significantly higher rates of complications, increased mortality, and longer length of stay in the malnourished groups. The level of malnourishment was also directly correlated with both severity and frequency of postoperative complications.

SURGICAL STRESS RESPONSE

There is a predictable series of physiologic changes that occur in response to surgical stress. The direct tissue injury from surgery leads to a widespread activation of the sympathetic nervous system as well as the hypothalamus-pituitary-adrenal axis, resulting in a surge of various stress hormones (ie, cortisol, adrenaline, adrenocorticotropic hormone, growth hormone) (**Fig. 1**).[4] Increased cortisol levels shift the body toward a hypermetabolic and catabolic state where all carbohydrates, fats, and proteins are metabolized to meet the body's increased energy expenditure. Furthermore, insulin resistance invariably develops in surgical patients and is directly related to the magnitude of the operation.[5] The stress response to surgery also results in impaired immune function via the preferential expression of

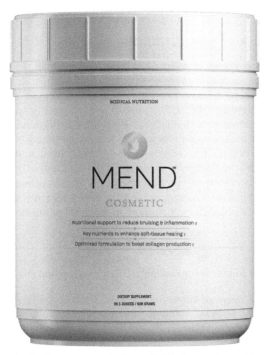

Fig. 1. Common products available for perioperative nutritional supplementation (Abbott Laboratories, Abbott Park, IL; MEND Nutrition Inc., New York, NY; Nestlé Health Science, Vevey, Switzerland).

T-helper 2 (Th2) lymphocytes. The Th2 cytokines stimulate the expression of arginase-1–producing myeloid-derived suppressor cells in lymphoid tissue. The arginine deficient state that ensues is thought to cause impaired lymphocyte function and thus results in impaired cell-mediated immunity.[6]

PERIOPERATIVE OPTIMIZATION

The "Enhanced Recovery After Surgery" (ERAS) pathways were developed as a multimodal approach to reduce patients' stress response to surgical procedures, maintain baseline body composition and organ function, and consequently improve outcomes.[7,8] Its benefits were validated in multiple studies, including a Cochrane meta-analysis that showed a reduction in overall complication rates and length of hospital stay when compared with conventional recovery strategies.[9] Amongst the various evidence-based interventions proposed, the ERAS pathway emphasizes the importance of screening for and addressing malnutrition in the preoperative period. Indeed, less than 40% of severely malnourished patients were appropriately identified and managed when assessed arbitrarily by surgeons.[10] The primary goals in nutritional rehabilitation are to optimize nutrient stores and metabolic reserve preoperatively in order to provide adequate buffer to compensate for the catabolic response of surgery and limit the negative impacts of preoperative malnutrition.[11] Jie and colleagues[10] showed a 50% reduction in overall complication rate amongst "severely malnourished" patients undergoing abdominal surgery who received appropriate preoperative nutrition.

NUTRITIONAL INTERVENTION

Nutritional support has evolved substantially over the years and there currently exists a wide variety of nutritional supplementation strategies that can be used clinically. The recent development of "immune-modulating diets" (IMD) has raised significant interest due to its proposed ability to reverse many of the immune-mediated changes seen after surgery.[6,12] These specialized diets consist of balanced nutritional formulations supplemented with specific nutrients meant to improve immune function and modulate inflammation. Immune-modulating nutrients commonly added include arginine, glutamine, omega-3 fatty acids, and antioxidants (ie, ascorbic acid and selenium). Their use was hypothesized to counter the generalized state of immunosuppression induced by surgery. Arginine has been found to stimulate T lymphocytes and thus improve cell-mediated immunity and decrease the risk of infection. Arginine may serve to directly replete the low levels induced from the preferential expression of Th2 lymphocytes. Glutamine is a direct source of energy for various cells involved in wound healing, such as lymphocytes and fibroblasts. It also serves as a critical antioxidant and helps cope with stress. A meta-analysis compared the impact of IMDs, in the perioperative period, on the clinical outcomes of patients undergoing elective surgery.[12] The use of specialized formulas with added arginine and fish oil reduced the risk of acquired infections (OR 0.49; 95% CI 0.39–0.62, $P<.0001$) and wound complications (OR 0.60; 95% CI 0.40–0.91, $P = .02$), while also shortening hospital length of stay (−3.03 days; 95% CI -3.43 to −2.64 days, $P<.0001$).[12] Most of the studies (n = 17/21) included in the analysis were evaluating patients suffering from gastrointestinal malignancy. A separate systematic review looking at various preoperative nutritional support options in well-nourished surgical patients showed some morbidity benefits with the use of IMD. The use of IMD resulted in significantly lower rates of complications, particularly infective complications.[13]

NUTRITION IN PLASTIC SURGERY

The use of nutritional supplementation in cosmetic surgery has not been well established. Although cases of "severe malnutrition" would be unlikely, many of these patients may very likely suffer from marginal nutritional deficiencies that could be optimized in preparation for surgery. Indeed, food consumption surveys are demonstrating inadequate intake of essential vitamins and minerals in current diets, with up to 70% of adults in the United States not meeting their daily nutrient requirements.[14,15] Incorporating nutritional counseling in our surgical practice is crucial, as poor nutrition is one of the few modifiable risk factors for poor wound healing. Other notable benefits of nutritional supplementation on surgical outcomes are the reduction of oxidative stress, the impact on immune function, and the reduction in bruising and swelling. Taking a more proactive approach to managing perioperative nutrition could also provide physicians with the opportunity to ensure that contraindicated supplements and herbal remedies are appropriately discontinued before surgery. There has been a fascinating growth in the use of alternative and complementary medicines over the past few decades; high rates of herbal remedy use have been specifically reported in facial cosmetic surgery patients.[16] The obvious concern surrounding the use of such supplements is regarding their unknown drug-drug interactions, increased bleeding risk, and cardiovascular and sedative effects. More concerning is the fact that up to 70% of patients do not explicitly report the use of herbal supplements to their health care providers.[17] Patients undergoing cosmetic procedures are generally motivated patients who are particularly invested in their health and perioperative care. The facial plastic surgery patients with cosmetic concerns are willing to invest in themselves and ensure that they have the most optimal recovery possible. It is our responsibility to provide these patients with clear nutritional guidance in order to optimize surgical outcomes.

SPECIFIC BENEFICIAL COMPONENTS FOR IDEAL SUPPLEMENTATION

Ideal nutrients and supplements for facial plastic surgery patients are reviewed (**Table 1**):

- **Vitamin A**: vitamin A is required for epithelial and bone tissue development, cellular differentiation, and immune system function.[18] Vitamin A supplementation in animal studies has been shown to improve collagen synthesis and cross-linking, leading to increased wound strength.[17,19] Other benefits include reversing the steroid-induced inhibition of cutaneous and fascial wound healing.[20] Vitamin A supplementation of 25,000 IU daily before and after elective surgery has been recommended.[21] Short-term supplementation seems to be safe for most nonpregnant patients, as toxicities are usually reported with chronic ingestion of more than 50,000 IU daily.[22]
- **Vitamin C (ascorbic acid)**: vitamin C is an essential cofactor for the synthesis of collagen and other organic components of the intracellular matrix of various connective tissues (ie, bone, skin, capillary wall, etc.). Ascorbic acid has also been shown to enhance neutrophil function, increase angiogenesis, and act as a powerful antioxidant. Vitamin C is necessary in the inflammatory phase of wound healing, as it facilitates neutrophil function. It is also necessary in the proliferating and remodeling phases through its ability to synthesize collagen. The acute stress from surgery has been shown to result in decreased plasma levels of vitamin C, thus supporting the use of routine supplementation. Its safe toxicity profile, combined with its theoretic impact on collagen synthesis, oxidative stress

Table 1
Summary of nutritional benefits associated with common supplements

Ingredients	Tissue Healing	Reduce Bruising/ Inflammation	Collagen Production	Skin Health
Hydrolyzed collagen		X	X	X
Arnica		X		
Protein complex	X			
BCAA complex	X			
L-glutamine	X			
HMB	X			
Bioflavonoid mix	X			X
Arginine	X		X	
Vitamin B complex	X			
Selenium		X		
Vitamin C	X		X	X
Calcium	X		X	
Magnesium	X	X		
Vitamin A			X	X
Fructooligosaccharide		X		
Vitamin D3		X		X
Sodium				
Zinc	X			
Copper	X			X
Iron	X			
Manganese				X
Echinacea purpurea		X		X
Prebiotic blend				
Bromelain	X	X		

reduction, and immunomodulation makes vitamin C an ideal supplement in the perioperative period. Vitamin C supplementation of 1 to 2 g daily has been recommended, from wound onset until healing is complete.[21]

- **Zinc**: zinc is an essential trace mineral for DNA synthesis, cell division, and protein synthesis. It is thus necessary during the anabolic phases of wound healing. It is also required for the activity of more than 300 enzymes throughout the body. Zinc deficiency has been associated with poor wound healing and decreased wound strength in animal studies.[23] The routine supplementation of zinc in low doses (ie, 15–30 mg daily) may help optimize wound healing in patients with marginal deficiencies.

- **Bromelain**: bromelain consists of a proteolytic enzyme derived from the pineapple plant and is thought to have strong antiinflammatory properties. Studies in the late 1960s demonstrated improved healing as well as reduced edema, pain, and bruising following surgery.[24,25] Seltzer[26] investigated its use in patients undergoing rhinoplasty and found prolonged ecchymosis and swelling in the placebo group (ie, 7 vs 2 days). Bromelain has also peaked surgeons' interest due to its reported ability to increase the resorption rate of hematomas.[27]

- **Protein**: adequate protein intake is essential for all phases of normal wound healing. Protein deficiency has resulted in decreased wound strength in animal and human studies. Although minor surgery may not significantly increase a patient's protein requirements, maintaining adequate protein levels should avoid any protein-related wound-healing issues.

- **Arginine**: arginine is a nonessential amino acid that plays a key role in protein synthesis as well as immune function. Arginine has been found to stimulate T lymphocytes and thus improve cell-mediated immunity and decrease the risk of infection. The supplementation of arginine in surgical patients has led to improvement in wound healing and immune responsiveness.[28]

- **Glutamine**: glutamine is a direct source of energy for various cells involved in wound healing such as lymphocytes and fibroblasts. It also serves as a critical antioxidant and helps cope with the stress response. Its benefits have mainly been shown in critically ill patients.
- **Arnica montana**: derived from a mountain flower, this homeopathic entity has been compounded into both topical and ingestible formulations. Reported benefits of oral Arnicare tablets include reduction in swelling, bruising, and postoperative pain.[29,30] Ideal daily dosing is 200 C or greater.
- **Hydrolyzed collagen**: collagen is critical for maintaining healthy skin, joints, and blood vessel wall integrity. Although the mechanism remains unclear, researchers have shown increased levels of collagen in the skin and bloodstream following oral intake of hydrolyzed collagen; this was associated with improved skin aging.[31,32] Furthermore, osteoarthritis researchers have identified benefits in chondrocyte function and reduced pain symptoms associated with daily oral consumption of hydrolyzed collagen, supporting the notion of increased bone and cartilage health.[33]

THE CURRENT LANDSCAPE

Several meal-replacement and premade "shake" type products are currently available in the market, most notably being Boost and Ensure (see **Fig. 1**). These products provide a broad spectrum of vitamins and nutrients for the generally malnourished individual. There are also several companies that are creating a blend of their proprietary ingredients and nutrients into supplements for perioperative consumption. MEND Cosmetic (www.mend.me), created by the senior author (AJA), is one such product and has been specially formulated to target the optimization of wound healing following cosmetic surgery procedures. The primary advantage of all these products is that it allows patients to assume a "one-stop-shopping" approach to achieving ideal pre- and postoperative surgical nutrition, while avoiding any supplements that may be detrimental to surgical outcomes.

SUMMARY

Malnutrition has been shown to be a modifiable risk factor for increased morbidity and mortality in patients undergoing major surgery. The current guidelines advocate for routine nutritional assessment in surgical patients and supports nutritional rehabilitation in malnourished individuals. Despite mounting evidence supporting perioperative nutrition, there continues to be a gap in knowledge and interest within the surgical community. Incorporating nutritional interventions in the perioperative care of cosmetic surgery patients may help correct subclinical dietary deficiencies, accelerate recovery and improve surgical outcomes. Further studies are required to determine the ideal timing and composition of perioperative nutritional supplementation. Objective measures of surgical outcomes, as well as more subjective, patient-focused outcomes should be assessed.

REFERENCES

1. Shils ME, Shike M. Modern nutrition in health and disease. Philadelphia: Lippincott Williams & Wilkins; 2006.
2. Schneider SM, Veyres P, Pivot X, et al. Malnutrition is an independent factor associated with nosocomial infections. Br J Nutr 2004;92(1):105–11.
3. Kuzu MA, Terzioglu H, Genc V, et al. Preoperative nutritional risk assessment in predicting postoperative outcome in patients undergoing major surgery. World J Surg 2006;30(3):378–90.
4. Moor D, Aggarwal G, Quiney N. Systemic response to surgery. Surgery 2017;35. https://doi.org/10.1016/j.mpsur.2017.01.013.
5. Thorell A, Nygren J, Ljungqvist O. Insulin resistance: a marker of surgical stress. Curr Opin Clin Nutr Metab Care 1999;2(1):69–78.
6. Marik PE, Flemmer M. Immunonutrition in the surgical patient. Minerva Anestesiol 2012;78(3):336–42.
7. Steenhagen E. Enhanced recovery after surgery: it's time to change practice! Nutr Clin Pract 2016;31(1): 18–29.
8. Dort JC, Farwell DG, Findlay M, et al. Optimal perioperative care in major head and neck cancer surgery with free flap reconstruction: a consensus review and recommendations from the enhanced recovery after surgery society. JAMA Otolaryngol Head Neck Surg 2017;143(3):292–303.
9. Spanjersberg WR, Reurings J, Keus F, et al. Fast track surgery versus conventional recovery strategies for colorectal surgery. Cochrane Database Syst Rev 2011;(2):CD007635.
10. Jie B, Jiang ZM, Nolan MT, et al. Impact of preoperative nutritional support on clinical outcome in

abdominal surgical patients at nutritional risk. Nutrition 2012;28(10):1022–7.

11. West MA, Wischmeyer PE, Grocott MPW. Prehabilitation and nutritional support to improve perioperative outcomes. Curr Anesthesiol Rep 2017;7(4): 340–9.

12. Marik PE, Zaloga GP. Immunonutrition in high-risk surgical patients: a systematic review and analysis of the literature. JPEN J Parenter Enteral Nutr 2010;34(4):378–86.

13. Burden S, Todd C, Hill J, et al. Pre-operative nutrition support in patients undergoing gastrointestinal surgery. Cochrane Database Syst Rev 2012;(11): CD008879.

14. Block G. Dietary guidelines and the results of food consumption surveys. Am J Clin Nutr 1991;53: 356S–7S.

15. Kant AK, Schatzkin A. Consumption of energy dense, nutrient-poor foods by the U.S. population: effect on nutrient profiles. J Am Coll Nutr 1994;13: 285–91.

16. Zwiebel SJ, Lee M, Alleyne B, et al. The incidence of vitamin, mineral, herbal, and other supplement use in facial cosmetic patients. Plast Reconstr Surg 2013;132(1):78–82.

17. Greenwald DP, Sharzer LA, Padawer J, et al. Zone II flexor tendon repair: effects of vitamins A, E, beta-carotene. J Surg Res 1990;49:98–102.

18. MacKay D, Miller AL. Nutritional support for wound healing. Altern Med Rev 2003;8(4):359–77.

19. Seifter E, Crowley LV, Rettura G, et al. Influence of vitamin A on wound healing in rats with femoral fracture. Ann Surg 1975;181(6):836–41.

20. Ehrlich HP, Hunt TK. Effects of cortisone and vitamin A on wound healing. Ann Surg 1968;167:324–8.

21. Levenson SM, Demetrio AA. Metabolic factors. In: Cohen IK, Diegelmann RF, Linblad WJ, editors. Wound healing: biochemical and clinical aspects. Philadelphia: WB Saunders Co; 1992. p. 264.

22. Biesalski HK. Comparative assessment of the toxicology of vitamin A and retinoids in man. Toxicology 1989;57(2):117–61.

23. Agren MS, Franzen L. Influence of zinc deficiency on breaking strength of 3-week-old skin incisions in the rat. Acta Chir Scand 1990;156:667–70.

24. Tassman G, Zafran J, Zayon G. A double-blind crossover study of plant proteolytic enzyme in oral surgery. J Dent Med 1965;20:51–4.

25. Howat RC, Lewis GD. The effect of bromelain therapy on episiotomy wounds – a double blind controlled clinical trial. J Obstet Gynaecol Br Commonw 1972;79:951–3.

26. Seltzer AP. Minimizing post-operative edema and ecchymoses by the use of an oral enzyme preparation (bromelain): a controlled study of 53 rhinoplasty cases. Eye Ear Nose Throat Mon 1962;41:813–7.

27. Woolf RM, Snow JW, Walker JH, et al. Resolution of an artificially induced hematoma and the influence of a proteolytic enzyme. J Trauma 1965;5:491–8.

28. Barbul A, Lazarou SA, Efron DT, et al. Arginine enhances wound healing and lymphocyte immune responses in humans. Surgery 1990;108:331–6.

29. Iannitti T, Morales-Medina JC, Bellavite P, et al. Effectiveness and safety of Arnica montana in post-surgical setting, pain and inflammation. Am J Ther 2016;23(1):e184–97.

30. Lee HS, Yoon HY, Kim IH, et al. The effectiveness of postoperative intervention in patients after rhinoplasty: a meta-analysis. Eur Arch Otorhinolaryngol 2017;274(7):2685–94.

31. Yazaki M, Ito Y, Yamada M, et al. Oral ingestion of collagen hydrolysate leads to the transportation of highly concentrated Gly-Pro-Hyp and its hydrolyzed form of Pro-Hyp into the bloodstream and skin. J Agric Food Chem 2017;65(11):2315–22.

32. Dar QA, Schott EM, Catheline SE, et al. Daily oral consumption of hydrolyzed type 1 collagen is chondroprotective and anti-inflammatory in murine post-traumatic osteoarthritis. PLoS One 2017;12(4): e0174705.

33. Czajka A, Kania EM, Genovese L, et al. Daily oral supplementation with collagen peptides combined with vitamins and other bioactive compounds improves skin elasticity and has a beneficial effect on joint and general wellbeing. Nutr Res 2018;57: 97–108.

Platelet-Rich Plasma for Skin Rejuvenation
Facts, Fiction, and Pearls for Practice

Grace Lee Peng, MD

KEYWORDS

- Platelet-rich plasma • Microneedling • Collagen induction • Platelet gel • Skin rejuvenation
- Facial rejuvenation • Wrinkles • Acne scars

KEY POINTS

- Use of platelet-rich plasma in plastic surgery.
- Facial plastic surgery and platelet-rich plasma use.
- Microneedling and platelet-rich plasma.
- Microneedling for acne scars.

INTRODUCTION
Platelet Function in Hemostasis and Wound Healing

Platelets are an important part of hemostasis as well as the process of wound healing. There are 3 stages to wound healing: inflammatory, proliferative, and remodeling.[1–4] During inflammation, the goal is for hemostasis and the initiation of the wound-healing process.

With tissue injury, platelets come in direct contact with and aggregate at the site of damaged blood vessels.[5] Tissue injury also leads to platelet activation, which in turn leads platelets to release biologically active proteins and growth factors that promote wound healing. This includes platelet-derived growth factor, transforming growth factor-β, fibroblast growth factor, epidermal growth factor, keratinocyte growth factor, and vascular endothelium growth factor, among others.[6,7] In addition, adhesion molecules, such as fibronectin and vitronectin, scaffolding proteins, such as fibrinogen, and other molecules responsible for intercellular binding and communication, are stimulated. Together, they promote connective tissue healing, epithelial development, angiogenesis, and deposition of collagen matrix[6,7] (Table 1).

Platelet-Rich Plasma

Platelet-rich plasma (PRP) is autologous blood plasma with a concentration of platelets well above baseline.[8–10] The usual concentration of platelets in the blood is approximately 150,000 to 400,000 platelets per cubic microliter.[1,8] PRP contains 4 to 7 times the physiologic concentration of platelets.[11,12] PRP is prepared by centrifugation of blood drawn from the patient before any procedure or surgery.[11]

The whole blood, once drawn, needs to have an anticoagulant to prevent clotting. Most PRP kits come with venipuncture tubes that already contain an anticoagulant. This anticoagulant is most often citrate, which will bind to the calcium ions, thus disrupting the coagulation cascade. In the anticoagulated state, the blood is stable for up to 8 hours.[9,13]

The next step in the processing of the PRP is centrifugation and subsequent separation of blood components (red blood cells, white blood cells and platelet-poor plasma, and PRP). In most cases, manufacturers will have their own centrifuges, which lead to differential centrifugation and yield a higher concentration of platelets and a cleaner separation of blood components.[8] To enhance this, many venipuncture tubes come

No financial disclosures.
Facial Plastic and Reconstructive Surgery, 120 South Spalding Drive, Suite 301, Beverly Hills, CA 90212, USA
E-mail address: drpeng@graceleepengmd.com

Table 1
Platelet growth factors and their mechanism of action

Growth Factors Released by Platelets	Mechanism
Platelet-derived growth factor	Initiates connective tissue healing Increases mitogenesis and angiogenesis Enhances collagen synthesis
Transforming growth factor-β	Increases chemotaxis Stimulates deposition of collagen matrix
Fibroblast growth factor	Stimulates angiogenesis Stimulate proliferation of myoblasts Promotes migration of fibroblasts
Epidermal growth factor	Increases proliferation of mesenchymal cells Increases proliferation of epithelial cells Enhances potentiation of other growth factors Stimulates differentiation of epithelial cells
Keratinocyte growth factor	Stimulates epithelialization
Vascular endothelium growth factor	Increases vascular permeability Enhances endothelial cell migration/proliferation Promotes collagen deposition

with various types of gel separators, which provide a gradient and allows for ease of separation during centrifugation.[14,15] After centrifugation, the platelet concentration in the plasma is considered PRP. However, there is no evidence the concentration of platelets is proportional to efficacy[16,17] (**Fig. 1**).

At this stage of preparation, PRP can be used immediately. Because the various components of commercial collecting venipuncture tubes and systems differ in their concentrations of platelets as well as the active nature of the platelets, there may or may not be a need for further activation.[18–20] Some studies show that calcium-based activation is needed because the initial calcium was inhibited with the anticoagulant.[6,21,22]

Regardless of the concentration of platelets in the PRP, or the activation of the PRP after processing, the concentration of growth factors and biologically active proteins secreted by each individual will undoubtedly vary. This is due to not only each patient's own responses but also the number of platelets that are active. Currently, there are not many studies measuring the amount of growth factors as related to the concentration of PRP.

Clinical Use

PRP has been used for orthopedic indications, wound healing, facial skin rejuvenation, and hair restoration.[23,24] In studies for facial skin rejuvenation, PRP has been shown to improve texture, wrinkles, and facial volume.[24]

Application for Skin Rejuvenation

Use of platelet-rich plasma in conjunction with microneedling

Microneedling is the result of multiple, often oscillating needles causing damage to the skin, which then induces the skin itself to repair by collagen stimulation. The needles in microneedling devices are extremely fine and can penetrate up to a depth of 3 mm.[25] They reach the papillary and reticular dermis in a purely mechanical way. Therefore, there is preservation of stratum corneum and the epidermal barrier function, leading to the lack of scarring.[26,27] Microneedling also does not carry with it thermal injury and necrosis, thus making it safe for patients of all skin types and Fitzpatrick classification[10,26] (**Table 2**).

However, this trauma alone can activate the healing process. Immediately following the injury, fibroblasts inundate the region for wound healing, stimulating endothelial cells and starting the process of neoangiogenesis, and elastin and collagen production.[27–29] Commonly termed collagen induction therapy, microneedling has been used to improve the appearance of acne scarring, skin discoloration, melasma, fine lines, wrinkles, and facial scars.[29,30] When used in conjunction with PRP, its effects can be potentiated and can help improve skin elasticity.[26]

Immediately after the procedure, there will be redness from pinpoint areas of minimal bleeding. Redness usually does not last long, with most patients having minimal redness after the first 1 to 2 days. Some patients with more sensitive skin

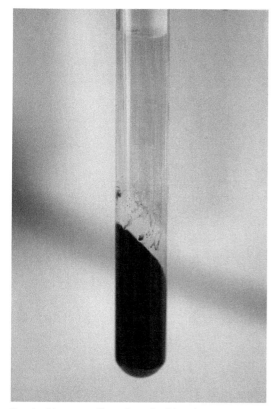

Fig. 1. After centrifugation, the blood separates into its various layers with the bottom layer being the red blood cells, the middle layer being the white blood cells, and the upper layer being the PRP.

may have more prolonged redness. Of note, areas of thinner skin, such as periorbital regions, over the upper nasal dorsum, and areas of the forehead may have some increased chances of localized bruising.

Use of platelet-rich plasma as facial injection
PRP is commonly injected to the face and neck to help increase facial volume through collagen

Table 2
Microneedling devices and their depth of penetration

Name of Pen	Depth (mm)
Collagen PIN	3.0
Cosmo Pen	2.5
CytoPen	2.5
DermaPen	2.5
MD Needle Pen	2.5
MD Pen	2.8
MesopenMD	2.0
Micropen	2.5
Rejuvapen	2.5

stimulation.[18,31,32] This injection can be either intradermal or subdermal, or a combination of the two. PRP injections have been shown to improve the skin color and texture as well as the depth of fine lines and wrinkles through an increase of dermal collagen.[18,27,31] However, given the depth of injection, there is no ability for topical numbing, and there are higher reports of pain and discomfort during the procedure. In addition, there may be increased downtime from bruising and some swelling.[33,34]

In general, these treatments are done at 4- to 6-week intervals and repeated at least 3 to 5 times, or until the desired result is achieved. Additional procedures for maintenance are performed in a timeline that is spaced out for maintenance (**Figs. 2** and **3C**).

PEARLS FOR PRACTICE

Numbing the patient before the procedure is important, because it allows for a pleasant experience. Topical numbing cream should be comprehensive, extending to all areas where microneedling will be performed. For example, the topical numbing should extend all the way to the edge of the hairline as well as to the edge of the tragus, if it is to be treated. Treated areas can also include the neck and décolleté. Topical numbing cream comes in a variety of forms,

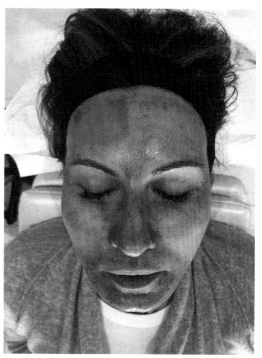

Fig. 2. Redness immediately after procedure is similar to that of a medium sunburn.

A

B

C

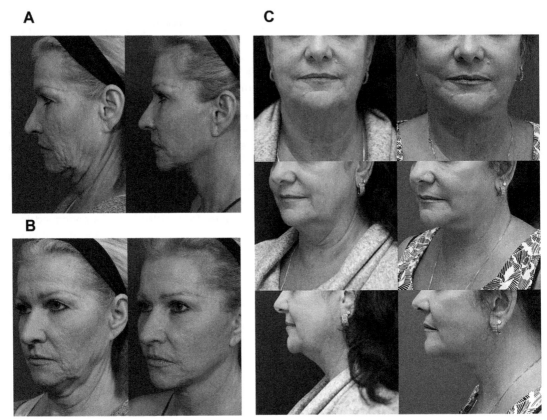

Fig. 3. (*A*) Microneedling performed 3 times spaced 1 month apart improved the appearance of ice pick acne scars, fine lines, and pores in this 60-year-old woman. (*B*) Microneedling performed 4 times spaced 1 month apart improved the active cystic acne as well as acne scars, and pore size in this 40-year-old woman. (*C*) Facial PRP injections in the midface performed 3 times spaced over 6 months as well as microneedling performed 2 times during those 6 months helped to improve the skin discoloration, fine lines, and the midfacial volume. This patient had also had a facelift, although the midface region was not entered during the facelift.

although the author has found a compounded ointment of lidocaine (10%), prilocaine (10%), and phenylephrine (0.25%) to be the most efficacious. Patients can be topically numbed immediately on arrival to the office for a duration of 45 to 60 minutes. During this time, they can also have their blood drawn in order to save time. These procedures add to office efficiency, because numbing can be done concurrently while waiting for the blood to be spun and processed.

Microneedling for various areas should be done at different depths, because the skin of the face, neck, and chest varies in its thickness. Each individual, their skin texture, and sebaceous quality should be taken into account, with patients with thicker skin able to have microneedling performed at deeper depths (**Fig. 4**).

Typically, to treat acne scars and other scars, the depth should range from 2.5 to 3 mm. However, areas of facial skin, such as the periorbital, upper nasal dorsal, and forehead areas, should be treated with depths of 0.5 to 1.5 mm, because of its thinner and more sensitive skin nature. Multiple passes in various directions should be used to ensure even treatment. As the needles oscillate, they will automatically puncture the skin to the desired depth, and additional pressure does not need to be used while using microneedling devices. It is important to avoid additional pressure and dragging the device along the skin, because that can cause deeper line injuries, irregularity, and unevenness.

Platelet-Rich Plasma Injection

Microneedling with PRP and injections of PRP can be combined during the same treatment. For most patients, microneedling will help the overall skin texture, whereas injections will further help collagen stimulation from the deeper tissues, helping to improve volume (**Fig. 5**).

Use of small needles such as a 32- or a 34-gauge needle will help with discomfort during

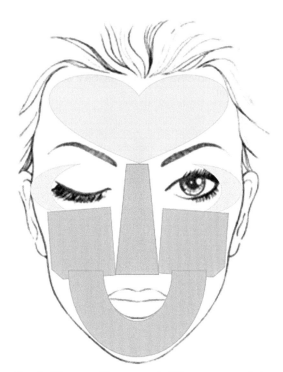

Fig. 4. Microneedling around different areas of the face should be performed at different depths and depends on the skin texture of each patient. Forehead: 1 to 1.5 mm; periorbital: 0.5 to 1 mm; face: 1.5 to greater than 2 mm; nasal skin, especially over the upper dorsum: 0.5 to 1 mm; neck and décolleté: 0.5 to 1.5 mm.

the procedure. Slow injection is recommended during the procedure, because this helps to overcome the mild burning sensation that may be experienced. Also, the use of an ice roller or

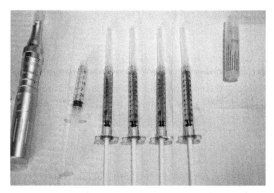

Fig. 5. Setup of a microneedling tray (from left to right): microneedling pen and single-use tip; PRP in a 3-cc syringe to be used while microneedling; PRP in 1-cc syringes with a 32-gauge needle for injection into the deeper dermis; hyaluronic acid for the patient to use at postprocedure day 1.

vibration device can improve patient comfort during the procedure. In general, given that there is a higher chance of bruising with injections of PRP, as opposed to microneedling with topical application, it is recommended that patients refrain from taking any blood thinners a few days before the procedure.

Reactivation of Herpes Simplex Virus and Prophylaxis

Patients with a history of cold sores should take prophylaxis with an antiviral before the procedure to prevent a flare-up after microneedling and PRP injections. Any procedure that causes trauma to the skin carries with it the potential of reactivation of the herpes simplex virus (HSV). With microneedling and PRP injections, it is possible that the tissue manipulation and the inflammatory reaction can reactivate the HSV. Although this is more likely after ablative procedures, it can be devastating to a patient coming in for what they expected to be a minimal-downtime, elective, skin rejuvenation procedure.[35,36] Recommendations for prophylaxis include any patient with the following:

1. Previous outbreak after a procedure
2. Multiple herpetic outbreaks a year
3. Lip augmentation and subsequent outbreak
4. Facial resurfacing procedures (medium or deep peels, fractional lasers, microneedling)
5. Immunocompromised state[37]

There are no evidence-based studies comparing the prophylactic efficacy of acyclovir, valacyclovir, and famciclovir for these aesthetic patients. However, there are commonly recommended dosages, including acyclovir 400 mg twice daily (or 3 times for those at high risk) or valacyclovir 500 mg daily (or twice daily if high risk).[37] Antiviral medication is usually started the day before or the day of the procedure and for an additional 5 to 7 days.[38]

Despite the potentially beneficial properties of PRP, there are currently no studies that show whether PRP use in conjunction with a procedure, such as microneedling, will affect HSV reactivation. Awareness of cold sore reoccurrence and minimizing the HSV reactivation are important to prevent postprocedure complications.

POSTPROCEDURAL RECOMMENDATIONS

Patients should always avoid direct sunlight immediately after and for at least 2 weeks following the procedure. Sun protection should always be used. Hydration of the skin is also important and can be achieved with a variety of hyaluronic acid serums.

In addition, pairing the microneedling with microdermabrasion 7 to 10 days after the procedure can help to remove some of the dead skin cells and with the efficacy of cellular turnover. Intense hydration, such as with a Hydrafacial, at the same time, can also help to enhance results.

Contraindications to Use of Platelet-Rich Plasma

Although the use of PRP has a relatively low side-effect profile, there are some contraindications for its use.[39] Absolute contraindications include platelet dysfunction syndrome, hemodynamic instability, chronic liver disease, local infection at the site of the procedure, septicemia, hypofibrinogenemia, and anticoagulant use.[19,39]

Relative contraindications include use of nonsteroidal anti-inflammatory drugs within 48 hours of the procedure, corticosteroids injection in the area of treatment within a month before the procedure, systemic corticosteroids, tobacco use, recent illness and fever, cancer hemoglobin less than 10 g/dL, or thrombocytopenia with a platelet count less than $10^5/\mu L$, and autoimmune conditions not associated with thrombocytopenia.[39]

In general, in an outpatient setting, most of these contraindications are rare due to the overall health of patients seeking elective skin rejuvenation procedures. However, asking about platelet dysfunction, bleeding issues, recent illnesses, and localized infections is important.

SUMMARY

Being a product of autologous blood, PRP is relatively safe for use in facial rejuvenation procedures. It is always recommended that handling patient blood products be done in a safe and sterile manner to prevent contamination, especially in situations wherein there are multiple patients all receiving treatments at the same time.

PRP appears to have efficacy in the management of acne scarring, and when combined with microneedling, has improved results as compared with microneedling alone and injection alone.

Currently, there are no set guidelines about obtaining and processing PRP to yield the most efficacious plasma solution or platelet concentration. Variables that may affect the efficacy of PPR include the volume of blood obtained, anticoagulant used, the speed and time for centrifugation, and activating agents.

Clinical studies that compare these various forms will help provide better insight as to which PRP is better suited for various aesthetic purposes. Well-controlled, split-side treatments will be able to better define efficacy and minimize the inevitable intersubject variability.

Incorporating the use of PRP into any clinic and practice can help with patient retention, as well as conversion into other procedures, be it surgical or nonsurgical.

REFERENCES

1. Eppley BL, Pietrzak WS, Blanton M. Platelet-rich plasma: a review of biology and applications in plastic surgery. Plast Reconstr Surg 2006;118(6):147e–59e.
2. Anitua E, Andia I, Ardanza B, et al. Autologous platelets as a source of proteins for healing and tissue regeneration. Thromb Haemost 2004;91(1):4–15.
3. Andia I, Abate M. Platelet rich plasma: underlying biology and clinical correlates. Regen Med 2013;8:645–58.
4. Tischler M. Platelet rich plasma. The use of autologous growth factors to enhance bone and soft tissue grafts. N Y State Dent J 2002;68(3):22–4.
5. Cho EB, Park GS, Park SS, et al. Effect of platelet-rich plasma on proliferation and migration in human dermal fibroblasts. J Cosmet Dermatol 2018. [Epub ahead of print].
6. Bhanot S, Alex JC. Current applications of platelet gels in facial plastic surgery. Facial Plast Surg 2002;18(1):27–33.
7. Liu Y, Kalén A, Risto O, et al. Fibroblast proliferation due to exposure to a platelet concentrate in vitro is pH dependent. Wound Repair Regen 2002;10(5):336–40.
8. Alves R, Grimalt R. A review of platelet-rich plasma: history, biology, mechanism of action, and classification. Skin Appendage Disord 2018;4(1):18–24.
9. Marx RE. Platelet-rich plasma (PRP): what is PRP and what is not PRP? Implant Dent 2001;10:225.
10. Shin M-K, Lee JH, Lee SJ, et al. Platelet-rich plasma combined with fractional laser therapy for skin rejuvenation. Dermatol Surg 2012;38(4):623–30.
11. Marx RE. Platelet-rich plasma: evidence to support its use. J Oral Maxillofac Surg 2004;62(4):489–96.
12. Leo MS, Kumar AS, Kirit R, et al. Systematic review of the use of platelet-rich plasma in aesthetic dermatology. J Cosmet Dermatol 2015;14(4):315–23.
13. Anderson NA, Pamphilon DH, Tandy NJ, et al. Comparison of platelet-rich plasma collection using the Haemonetics PCS and Baxter Autopheresis C. Vox Sang 1991;60(3):155–8.
14. Sclafani AP. Platelet-rich fibrin matrix for improvement of deep nasolabial folds. J Cosmet Dermatol 2010;9(1):66–71.
15. Redaelli A, Romano D, Marciano A. Face and neck revitalization with platelet-rich plasma (PRP): clinical outcome in a series of 23 consecutively treated patients. J Drugs Dermatol 2010;9(5):466–72.

16. Guidelines for the use of platelet rich plasma. The International Cellular Medical Society; 2014.

17. Graziani F, Ivanovski S, Cei S, et al. The in vitro effect of different PRP concentrations on osteoblasts and fibroblasts. Clin Oral Implants Res 2006;17:212–9.

18. Yuksel EP, Sahin G, Aydin F, et al. Evaluation of effects of platelet-rich plasma on human facial skin. J Cosmet Laser Ther 2014;16(5):206–8.

19. Marwah M, Godse K, Patil S, et al. Is there sufficient research data to use platelet-rich plasma in dermatology? Int J Trichol 2014;6(1):35–6.

20. Abdali H, Hadilou M. Treatment of nasolabial fold with subdermal dissection and autologous fat injection added with platelet-rich plasma. J Res Med Sci 2014;19(11):1110.

21. Man D, Plosker H, Winland-Brown JE. The use of autologous platelet-rich plasma (platelet gel) and autologous platelet-poor plasma (fibrin glue) in cosmetic surgery. Plast Reconstr Surg 2001; 107(1):229–39.

22. Marx RE, Carlson ER, Eichstaedt RM, et al. Platelet-rich plasma: growth factor enhancement for bone grafts. Oral Surg Oral Med Oral Pathol Oral Radiol Endod 1998;85(6):638–46.

23. Hsu WK, Mishra A, Rodeo SR, et al. Platelet-rich plasma in orthopaedic applications: evidence-based recommendations for treatment. J Am Acad Orthop Surg 2013;21(12):739–48.

24. Frautschi RS, Hashem AM, Halasa B, et al. Current evidence for clinical efficacy of platelet rich plasma in aesthetic surgery: a systematic review. Aesthet Surg J 2017;37(3):353–62.

25. Ramut L, Hoeksema H, Pirayesh A, et al. Microneedling: where do we stand now? A systematic review of the literature. J Plast Reconstr Aesthet Surg 2011; 71:1–14.

26. Asif M, Kanodia S, Singh K. Combined autologous platelet-rich plasma with microneedling verses microneedling with distilled water in the treatment of atrophic acne scars: a concurrent split-face study. J Cosmet Dermatol 2016;15(4):434–43.

27. El-Domyati M, Abdel-Wahab H, Hossam A. Microneedling combined with platelet-rich plasma or trichloroacetic acid peeling for management of acne scarring: a split-face clinical and histologic comparison. J Cosmet Dermatol 2018;17(1):73–83.

28. Orentreich DS, Orentreich N. Subcutaneous incisionless (subcision) surgery for the correction of depressed scars and wrinkles. Dermatol Surg 1995;21:543–9.

29. Majid I. Microneedling therapy in atrophic facial scars: an objective assessment. J Cutan Aesthet Surg 2009;2:26–30.

30. Bharadwaj D. Collagen induction therapy with dermaroller. Community Based Med J 2012;1:35–7.

31. Kim DH, Je YJ, Kim CD, et al. Can platelet-rich plasma be used for skin rejuvenation? Evaluation of effects of platelet-rich plasma on human dermal fibroblast. Ann Dermatol 2011;23(4):424–31.

32. Willemsen JCN, van der Lei B, Vermeulen KM, et al. The effects of platelet-rich plasma on recovery time and aesthetic outcome in facial rejuvenation: preliminary retrospective observations. Aesthetic Plast Surg 2014;38(5):1057–63.

33. Cameli N, Mariano M, Cordone I, et al. Autologous pure platelet-rich plasma dermal injections for facial skin rejuvenation: clinical, instrumental, and flow cytometry assessment. Dermatol Surg 2017;43(6): 826–35.

34. Gawdat HI, Hegazy RA, Fawzy MM, et al. Autologous platelet rich plasma: topical versus intradermal after fractional ablative carbon dioxide laser treatment of atrophic acne scars. Dermatol Surg 2014; 40(2):152–61.

35. Beeson WH, Rachel JD. Valacyclovir prophylaxis for herpes simplex virus infection or infection recurrence following laser skin resurfacing. Dermatol Surg 2002;28(4):331–6.

36. Bisaccia E, Scarborough D. Herpes simplex virus prophylaxis with famciclovir in patients undergoing aesthetic facial CO2 laser resurfacing. Cutis 2003; 72(4):327–8.

37. King M. Prophylaxis and treatment of herpetic infections. J Clin Aesthet Dermatol 2017;10(1):E5–7.

38. Convery C. Aesthetic treatment and herpes simplex virus. Aesthetics Journal 2017. Available at: https://aestheticsjournal.com/feature/aesthetic-treatments-and-herpes-simplex-virus. Accessed January 2019.

39. Ranaweera A. Platelet rich plasma. Available at: https://www.dermnetnz.org/topics/platelet-rich-plasma-dermatological-applications/. Accessed January 20, 2019.

Relevant Topical Skin Care Products for Prevention and Treatment of Aging Skin

Sarmela Sunder, MD

KEYWORDS

• Aging skin • Skin care • Cosmeceuticals • Topical skin care • Antiaging

KEY POINTS

- UV radiation, DNA damage, free radical formation, and inflammation contribute to skin aging.
- Changes in cellular structure and physiology effect the changes on the skin that are perceived as aging skin.
- Retinoids are a group of extremely well-studied topicals that have shown to have beneficial effects on mild to moderate photodamaged skin.
- Ascorbic acid can improve the effects of photodamage by stimulating the production of procollagen and by improving appearance of fine lines and dyspigmentation.
- Glycolic acid products improve the appearance of skin by increasing cell turnover.

INTRODUCTION

Skin care and cosmeceuticals are quickly becoming an important part of a facial plastic surgery practice. The patient who invests in proper skin care before surgery can realize antiaging benefits, and the patient who invests in effective skin care after surgery can enjoy some improved outcomes in overall skin quality and appearance.

There are a myriad of options for cosmeceuticals that can leave the practitioner and patient equally confused as to their benefits, efficacy, and use. To understand the role of each topical skin care product, we must first understand the basics of skin anatomy and the mechanisms of skin aging.

FACTORS AFFECTING SKIN AGING

Several factors contribute to aging skin, specifically extrinsic factors and intrinsic factors, causing extrinsic aging and intrinsic aging, respectively. Extrinsic factors are the environmental causes of skin aging, such as UV light, infrared light, and radiation exposure. Sun exposure, air pollution, stress,

poor diet, inadequate nutrition, smoking, alcohol, drugs, excess sugar intake, and tanning beds have all been indicated as extrinsic contributions to aging.[1] Some articles cite that sun exposure contributes to up to 80% of facial aging.[2] The mechanism through which sun exposure plays a role in aging is through UV light causing direct DNA damage. UV light creates free radicals that cause oxidative stress. This process in turn releases and activates arachidonic acid that, when oxygenated by enzyme systems, lead to the formation of an important group of inflammatory mediators, the eicosanoids.[3] It is now recognized that eicosanoid release is fundamental to the inflammatory process, particularly leading to inflammation in the skin. UV exposure induces covalent bonds between nucleic acid pairs, forming thymine dimers.[4] These thymine dimers, in turn, alter the function of p53, a tumor suppressor gene. As a result of suppressing a tumor suppressor gene, the risk of skin cancer and skin aging are upregulated.[4]

Consumption of toxins (smoking, alcohol, drugs), UV radiation, free radical formation, pollution, and inflammation can all cause various types

Disclosure Statement: The author has nothing to disclose.
436 North Bedford Drive, Suite 103, Beverly Hills, CA 90210, USA
E-mail address: dr.sarmela.sunder@gmail.com

Facial Plast Surg Clin N Am 27 (2019) 413–418
https://doi.org/10.1016/j.fsc.2019.04.007
1064-7406/19/© 2019 Elsevier Inc. All rights reserved.

of cell component damage, which leads to aging changes in the skin. DNA damage (both nuclear and mitochondrial) and damage to cell membranes and related proteins can manifest significant changes in skin quality.[5]

The second class of aging is known as intrinsic aging. Intrinsic aging, also referred to as chronologic aging, is influenced by genetics and occurs as the result of cellular processes that occur over time.[6] Decreased function of fibroblasts and keratinocytes, cells critical for skin architecture, the accumulation of intracellular and extracellular of byproducts, mitochondrial damage, and the decreased function of sirtuins and telomeres, all contribute to the intrinsic aging of the skin. Sirtuins are proteins involved in regulating cellular processes, including the aging and death of cells and their resistance to stress.[5] In general, extrinsic aging occurs from a combination of multiple processes caused by free radicals, DNA damage, glycation, inflammation, and other actions of the immune system.

Skin that has aged owing to extrinsic factors is characterized by dyschromia and mottled discoloration in the form of sunspots, deep wrinkles, and evidence of epidermal atrophy.[7–9] In addition, the accumulation of amorphous elastin material with reduced elasticity, referred to as elastosis, is another characteristic of extrinsically aged skin.[7,8] Finally, collagen fibers in extrinsically aged skin become thickened, fragmented, and more soluble.[10,11]

In contrast, intrinsic aging is associated with the natural deterioration of skin components, a decreased ability of cell turnover (known as senescence), and structural changes to subcutaneous tissue that occur over time.[7] Characteristics of intrinsically aged skin include laxity, fine wrinkling, and deepened expression lines. However, the skin remains smooth and unblemished with typical geometric patterns. Intrinsically aged skin also has evidence of atrophy with flattened epidermal rete ridges.[7–9] In the dermal extracellular matrix, collagen type I is lost and overall collagen levels decrease.[9] On a more cellular level, intrinsic skin aging displays a decreased ability to repair damage and has fewer fibroblasts and mast cells.[7–9]

The effects of these extrinsic and intrinsic factors lead to dermal atrophy, decreased collagen, decreased elasticity of the skin, increased melanogenesis, and the development of dyschromias.

Skin Structure and Changes in Aging

The epidermis is composed of keratinocytes laid out in 5 layers: the stratum basale, stratum spinosum, stratum granulosum, stratum lucidum, and stratum corneum. Damage to any layer of the epidermis can lead to increased skin aging. The stratum corneum serves as a protective skin barrier. This layer has cross-linked proteins for strength and antioxidants to protect it from oxidative damage and free radicals.[10]

These corneocytes are embedded in a lipid matrix composed of ceramides, cholesterol, and fatty acids. The stratum corneum functions as a barrier to protect the underlying tissue from infection, dehydration, chemicals, and mechanical stress. Desquamation, the process of cell shedding from the surface of the stratum corneum, balances proliferating keratinocytes that form in the stratum basale. These cells migrate up through the epidermis toward the surface in a journey that takes approximately 14 days.[11,12] In addition, there is a double layer lipid membrane that prevents water evaporation.

The dermis, the layer deep to the epidermis, is composed of fibroblasts, which are responsible for the production of collagen (imparts strength), elastin (confers elasticity), and various glycosaminoglycans, such as hyaluronic acid, heparan sulfate, and dermatan sulfate (provides volume and support for cell-to-cell communication.)[11,12]

SUNSCREEN

The UV rays that we are exposed to consist of UVB and UVA photons. UVA rays are longer in wavelength and penetrate into deeper layers of skin, producing free radicals and contributing to premature skin aging. UVB rays are shorter in wavelength and do not penetrate as deeply into the skin.[13] These rays can cause significant DNA damage and are the primary contributors to skin cancer. It is well-accepted that routine sunscreen use helps to block the effects of this UV radiation. Various antioxidants also have protective effects against DNA damage caused by UV radiation and play a role in DNA repair.

Sunscreen with an SPF of at least 30 has been proven to have antiaging effects, as well as protective benefits against skin cancer.[14,15] Sunscreen prevents the UV rays from causing damage to the underlying skin. Some products absorb UV light, whereas others have inorganic pigments that absorb, scatter, and/or reflect UV rays.[14] There is a well-established consensus on the benefits of sunscreen use for photoprotection. The American Academy of Dermatology recommends that a broad spectrum sunscreen with an SPF of 30 or higher be used.

RETINOIDS

The benefits of retinoids, in reversing and preventing aging changes, have been well-documented in the literature. Retinoids achieve their effects in the skin through regulated gene expression, binding to retinoid acid receptors with DNA binding domains. Through these mechanisms, they contribute to procollagenesis and increase fibroblast growth. Retinoids also inhibit the formation of metalloproteinases, which degrade cellular matrices.[16–18] Studies have demonstrated that in concentrations of 0.02% or higher, retinoids have been shown to improve mild to moderate photodamage, fine and coarse wrinkles, ephelides, pigmentation, and overall skin texture.[16,17]

Some side effects of retinoids, which can lead to noncompliance, include irritation, erythema, scaling, and dryness. The majority of adverse effects have peak occurrence after 2 weeks of daily use and improve over time. The side effects are more common with a higher concentration of retinoid (0.1%) compared with the lower concentration (0.025%).[16,17] Some recommendations for reducing side effects and improving compliance include using a lubricating moisturizer before the application of retinoids and starting with a slow "ramp up" of the product application. For example, rather than starting application on a nightly basis, it may be recommended that patients start using it twice a week for 2 weeks, then advance the applications to every other night for 2 weeks, and finally advance the topical application of the retinoid to every night, as tolerated.

ALPHA HYDROXY ACIDS

Over the past 2 decades, alpha hydroxy acids (AHA) have gained increasing popularity as an ingredient in the antiaging armamentarium. The most commonly used AHAs are glycolic acid and lactic acid, although citric acid, malic acid, pyruvic acid, tartaric acid, and other AHAs have similar uses and function.[19] The benefits of AHAs have been known for many years, with evidence of historic figures using milk to wash the face and fruit puree as facial masks.

The most widely accepted theory of the mechanism of action of AHAs is that, through chelation, AHAs remove calcium ions from epidermal cell adhesions.[20] The resulting weakening of the intercellular adhesions has an exfoliating effect by causing the shedding of dead and dry skin cells.[21,22] In addition, the decreased calcium levels support further cell growth while slowing cell differentiation. This process allows for the reduced appearance of fine lines and wrinkles in the skin.[23] AHAs may also have a role in improving the hydration of the skin and lend to its plumpness, by effecting increased gene expression of collagen and hyaluronic acid in the dermis and epidermis.[21]

Over-the-counter formulations of AHAs are limited to 10%. Higher concentrations may be prescribed by medical offices and 40% AHA peels can be applied only by physicians. At concentrations of 25%, AHAs promote increased epidermal thickness and increased production of hyaluronic acid and collagen.[21]

VITAMIN C (ASCORBIC ACID)

Both oral and topical forms of ascorbic acid, better known as vitamin C, have been shown to impart beneficial effects on skin aging. In its topical form, vitamin C is an effective antioxidant, impeding free radical damage by both intracellularly and extracellularly neutralizing free radicals.[24] Vitamin C also promotes the synthesis of collagen through 2 studied mechanisms. First, ascorbic acid stimulates the formation of procollagen type I and type III and stimulates procollagen genes in fibroblasts. Second, ascorbic acid is a critical cofactor for several enzymes (including prolyl hydroxylase and lysyl hydroxylase) involved in collagen biosynthesis.[24]

In addition, topical application of ascorbic acid, in combination with vitamin E and ferulic acid, has been shown to decrease the formation of thymine dimers.[25] Thymine dimers can form as a result of exposure to UV radiation. When thymine absorbs UV rays, it becomes reactive with an adjacent thymine molecule in the DNA. This resultant dimer makes it impossible for RNA polymerase to properly read the DNA and thereby create an accurate mRNA, preventing the cell from creating the correct protein.

An abundance of thymine dimers, which cannot be repaired, cause the cells to die, as can be seen in the case of sunburns. In addition, thymine dimers can cause downstream effects, leading to malignant transformation of cells.[24,26]

A recent split face study by Xu and colleagues,[27] evaluating the topical application of 23% ascorbic acid demonstrated significant improvement in fine lines, surface roughness and dyspigmentation. Skin biopsies after topical application of ascorbic acid have shown an increase in collagen as well as an increased messenger RNA staining for type I collagen.[28]

GROWTH FACTORS

There are several growth factors that stimulate old keratinocytes and fibroblasts to increase function. Growth factors, such as vascular endothelial growth factor, epidermal growth factor, granulocyte-colony stimulating factor, platelet-derived growth factor, keratinocyte growth factor, and hepatocyte growth factor, have been shown to directly affect collagen biosynthesis.[8]

Human dermal growth factors and cytokines are important for collagen, elastin, and hyaluronic acid production. Changes in hyaluronic acid production and its degradation is associated with aging of the skin.[8] The balance of hyaluronic acid synthesis and metabolization is critical for extracellular matrix homeostasis. Specific growth factors that contribute to this interplay include transforming growth factor-β1, basic fibroblast growth factor, epidermal growth factor, and platelet-derived growth factor-BB. Through the upregulation of hyaluronic acid synthase expression, these factors play a role in skin fibroblast production of hyaluronic acid.[8,29,30] Supporting this finding is evidence that shows that fibroblasts treated with certain growth factors are able to incite healing and repair mechanisms in the skin, including the synthesis of the extracellular matrix and angiogenesis.[12]

Although studies have shown that topical applications of these growth factors and cytokines have clinically significant effects on skin rejuvenation, their relatively larger molecular weight poses a predicament. These growth factors and cytokines are typically greater than 15,000 Da, which hinders their ability to penetrate through the stratum corneum. In fact, in general, molecules larger than 500 Da have difficulty passing through the stratum corneum to reach the target keratinocytes in the stratum basal. Other sources of access include sweat glands, hair follicles, and compromised skin, such as the result of laser treatments or microneedling.

HEPARAN SULFATE

Heparan sulfate is a glycosaminoglycan that serves an important role in providing mechanical strength to the skin and occupies the space between collagen and elastin fibrils. It has functions in cell-to-cell communication and increases the cell's response to growth factors. Some specific functions of heparan sulfate include binding and protecting growth factors, effectively helping transport them to the appropriate target.

STEM CELLS

In general, the vast majority of cosmeceutical products that contain stem cells to date have not been proven to be particularly effective in preventing or treating skin aging. Most of the stem cell products on the market are derived from plant sources and are not able to function as human stem cells. In addition, these particles are usually too large to penetrate the stratum corneum to reach the keratinocytes. There is some promising evidence surrounding the idea of stimulating native stem cells, such as basal stem cells and hair follicle stem cells, in the skin. In specific, the LGR6+ hair follicle cells are critical in repopulating the epidermis after it is wounded, which actually stimulates these cells. When creating skin wounds, such as with a laser, peel, or needle puncture, neutrophils release defensin, a peptide that stimulates the LGR6+ cells to repopulate the epidermis. A topical form of defensin that penetrates into the hair follicles has demonstrated an ability to provide a smoother appearance to skin.[31,32]

PIGMENTATION

In recent years, tranexamic acid (trans-4-aminomethylcyclohexanecarboxylic acid) has been used as an agent to decrease pigmentation in melasma and UV-induced hyperpigmentation.[33–36] Tranexamic acid is an antifibrinolytic agent, which inhibits the plasmin/plasminogen pathway. It impedes the conversion of plasminogen to plasmin by inhibiting plasminogen activator through the formation of a reversible complex with plasminogen.[37] Maeda and colleagues[36] reported that UV-induced hyperpigmentation and pigmentation induced by topical application of arachidonic acid in guinea pigs was reduced by topical application of tranexamic acid in a dose-dependent manner. They suggest that, by inhibiting the binding of plasminogen to the keratinocyte, tranexamic acid inhibits UV-induced plasmin activity in keratinocytes. This eventually results in less free arachidonic acid and a decreased prostaglandin production, which in turn plays a role in hormone mediated melasma.

Topical skin care products that incorporate tranexamic acid have been shown to have promising effects as a treatment for melasma and pigmentation.[38,39]

Several studies have shown that topical use of tranexamic acid decreased epidermal pigmentation associated with melasma, as well as reversed melasma-related dermal changes, such as vessel number and increased numbers of mast cells.[39]

SUMMARY

Options for skin care are wide and varied, with newer products being introduced constantly. Therefore, it is important for the practitioner to have at least a basic understanding of the topical products that will impart beneficial results for aging skin. Educating patients to use products with scientifically proven benefits to prevent and/or treat aging changes of the skin will lead to better outcomes. At a minimum, patients should be encouraged to use daily sunscreen, a topical retinoid every night, and a topical antioxidant daily. Supplementing the routine skin care regimen with the use of AHAs, growth factors, heparin sulfate and defensins can be addressed individually. The use of exogenous stem cells, particularly those that are plant derived, do not have sufficient evidence to warrant recommending them at the current time.

REFERENCES

1. Baumann L. How to use oral and topical cosmeceuticals to prevent and treat skin aging. Facial Plast Surg Clin North Am 2018;26(4):407–13.
2. Uitto J. Understanding premature skin aging. N Engl J Med 1997;337:1463.
3. Samuelssen B. Arachidonic acid metabolism: role in inflammation. Z Rheumatol 1991;50(Suppl 1):3–6.
4. Tornaletti S, Pfeifer GP. Slow repair of pyrimidine dimers at p53 mutation hotspots in skin cancer. Science 1994;263:1436–8.
5. Glogau RG. Physiologic and structural changes associated with aging skin. Dermatol Clin 1997;15:555–9.
6. Thomas RJ, Dixon TK, Bhattacharyya TK. Effects of topicals on the aging skin process. Facial Plast Surg Clin North Am 2013;21(1):55–60.
7. Baumann L. Skin ageing and its treatment. J Pathol 2007;211(2):241–51.
8. Quan T, Fisher GJ. Role of age-associated alterations of the dermal extracellular matrix microenvironment in human skin aging: a mini-review. Gerontology 2015;61(5):427–34.
9. Khavkin J, Ellis DA. Aging skin: histology, physiology, and pathology. Facial Plast Surg Clin North Am 2011;19(2):229–34.
10. Bickers DR, Athar M. Oxidative stress in the pathogenesis of skin disease. J Invest Dermatol 2006;126:2562–75.
11. Mitra AK, Kwatra D, Vadlapudi AD. Drug delivery. Burlington (MA): Jones & Bartlett Learning; 2015. p. 285–6.
12. Ovaere P, Lippens S, Vandenabeele P, et al. The emerging roles of serine protease cascades in the epidermis. Trends Biochem Sci 2009;34(9):453–63.
13. Yaar M, Gilchrest BA. Photoageing, mechanism, prevention and therapy. Br J Dermatol 2007;157:874–87.
14. Stephens TJ, Herndon JH Jr, Colón LE, et al. The impact of natural sunlight exposure on the UVB-sun protection factor (UVB-SPF) and UVA protection factor (UVA-PF) of a UVA/UVB SPF 50 sunscreen. J Drugs Dermatol 2011;10(2):150–5.
15. Montagna W, Kirchner S, Carlisle K. Histology of sun-damaged human skin. J Am Acad Dermatol 1989;21(5 Pt 1):907–18.
16. Kang S, Voorhees J. Photoaging therapy with topical tretinoin: an evidence based analysis. J Am Acad Dermatol 1998;39(2):55–61.
17. Darlenski R, Surber C, Fluhr JW. Topical retinoids in the management of photo damaged skin: from theory to evidence-based practical approach. Br J Dermatol 2010;163(6):1157–65.
18. Fisher GL, Datta SC, Talwar HS, et al. Molecular basis of sun-induced premature skin aging and retinoid antagonism. Nature 1996;379:335–9.
19. Tran D, Townley JP, Barnes TM, et al. An antiaging skin care system containing alpha hydroxy acids and vitamins improves the biomechanical parameters of facial skin. Clin Cosmet Investig Dermatol 2015;8:9–17.
20. Ramos-e-Silva M, Celem LR, Ramos-e-Silva S, et al. Anti-aging cosmetics: facts and controversies. Clin Dermatol 2013;31(6):750–8.
21. Bernstein EF, Lee J, Brown DB, et al. Glycolic acid treatment increases type I collagen mRNA and hyaluronic acid content of human skin. Dermatol Surg 2001;27(5):429–33.
22. Smith WP. Epidermal and dermal effects of topical lactic acid. J Am Acad Dermatol 1996;35(3 Pt 1):187–95.
23. Rivers JK. The role of cosmeceuticals in antiaging therapy. Skin Therapy Lett 2008;13(8):5–9.
24. Boyera N, Galey I, Bernard BA. Effect of vitamin C and its derivatives on collagen synthesis and cross-linking by normal human fibroblasts. Int J Cosmet Sci 1998;20(3):151–8.
25. Pullar JM, Carr AC, Vissers MCM. The roles of vitamin C in skin health. Nutrients 2017;9(8):866.
26. Stamford NP. Stability, transdermal penetration, and cutaneous effects of ascorbic acid and its derivatives. J Cosmet Dermatol 2012;11(4):310–7.
27. Xu TH, Chen JZ, Li YH, et al. Split-face study of topical 23.8% L-ascorbic acid serum in treating photo-aged skin. J Drugs Dermatol 2012;11(1):51–6.
28. Fitzpatrick RE, Rostan EF. Double-blind half-face study comparing topical vitamin C and vehicle for rejuvenation of photodamage. Dermatol Surg 2002;28:231–6.
29. Fitzpatrick RE, Rostan EF. Reversal of photodamage with topical growth factors: a pilot study. J Cosmet Laser Ther 2003;5(1):25–34.
30. Aldag C, Nogueira Teixeira D, Leventhal PS. Skin rejuvenation using cosmetic products containing growth factors, cytokines, and matrikines: a review of the literature. Clin Cosmet Investig Dermatol 2016;9:411–9.
31. Ghieh F, Jurjus R, Ibrahim A, et al. The use of stem cells in burn wound healing: a review. Biomed Res Int 2015;2015:684084.

32. Lough D, Dai H, Yang M, et al. Stimulation of the follicular bulge LGR5+ and LGR6= stem cells with the gut-derived human alpha defense 5 results in decreased bacterial presence, enhanced wound healing, and hair growth from tissues devoid of adnexal structures. Plast Reconstr Surg 2013; 132(5):1159–71.

33. Lee JH, Park JG, Lim SH, et al. Localized intradermal microinjection of tranexamic acid for treatment of melasma in Asian patients: a preliminary clinical trial. Dermatol Surg 2006;32:626–31.

34. Li D, Shi Y, Li M, et al. Tranexamic acid can treat ultraviolet radiation-induced pigmentation in guinea pigs. Eur J Dermatol 2010;20:289–92.

35. Maeda K, Naganuma M. Topical trans-4 aminomethylcyclohexanecarboxylic acid prevents ultraviolet radiation-induced pigmentation. J Photochem Photobiol B 1998;47:136–41.

36. Maeda K, Tomita Y. Mechanism of the inhibitory effect of tranexamic acid on melanogenesis in cultured human melanocytes in the presence of keratinocyte-conditioned medium. J Health Sci 2007;53:389–96.

37. Dunn CJ, Goa KL. Tranexamic acid: a review of its use in surgery and other indications. Drugs 1999; 57:1005–32.

38. Kondou S, Okada Y, Tomita Y. Clinical study of effect of tranexamic acid emulsion on melasma and freckles. Skin Res 2007;6:309–15.

39. Na JI, Choi SY, Yang SH, et al. Effect of tranexamic acid on melasma: a clinical trial with histological evaluation. J Eur Acad Dermatol Venereol 2013;27: 1035–9.

Autologous Fat Harvest and Preparation for Optimal Predictable Outcomes

Christian H. Barnes, MD, Corey S. Maas, MD*

KEYWORDS

- Fat transfer • Adipocyte-derived stem cells • Mesenchymal stem cells

KEY POINTS

- Tissue harvesting and processing should be gentle to avoid unnecessary adipose destruction.
- The processing technique used should maximize the retention of MSCs for injection to aid in mitigation of the immune response to grafting and creation of a local environment maximizing adipocyte integration and differentiation.
- Donor site, processing technique, and portions of the processed tissue used for fat transfer can impact the chance of successful tissue transplantation.

 Video content accompanies this article at http://www.facialplastic.theclinics.com.

INTRODUCTION

Loss of facial volume by atrophy and inferior migration of facial fat pads, resorption of the bony skeleton, and thinning of the skin all work to diminish the fullness of the youthful face with aging. Surgeons using fat grafting to the face have been thwarted by variable and limited graft survival yielding less predictable results compared with the more predictable manufactured filler products, such as hyaluronic acid.[1] The trade off with less predictable, long-lasting results of fat compared with shorter acting but predictable hyaluronic acid fillers has relegated fat primarily to use in the larger fat pad regions of the face, such as the cheeks and temples. Fat grafting is also more invasive than hyaluronic acid fillers, because it requires harvesting from a donor site and is therefore often paired with other procedures, such as facelift.[2] Despite these limitations fat grafting remains a good treatment option for many patients with soft tissue deficiencies of the face and can engender high patient satisfaction if well understood.[3]

TISSUE COMPONENTS

The focus of fat transfer has long been about implanting living adipocytes from one region to another, but this focus has been shifting as the understanding of additional cell types, which interact with the transferred cells, increases. These additional cells are primarily the adipose-derived mesenchymal stem cells or medicinal signaling cells (MSCs). These cells, which are not fully pluripotent, are derived from pericytes residing along the microvasculature of the adipose tissue and are included in the stromal vascular tissue present in the donor tissue.[4] MSCs make up less than one-tenth of 1% of donor tissue in historically conventionally processed fat grafts.[5] Despite the small number of cells, they are active in orchestrating the inflammatory milieu at the donor site. These MSCs release signaling molecules integral in local immunomodulation, antiapoptosis, angiogenesis, antifibrosis, chemoattraction, cell growth, and progenitor differentiation.[6,7] These functions help support the transplanted cells in their new

Disclosure Statement: The authors have nothing to disclose.
Facial Plastic and Reconstructive Surgery, The Maas Clinic, 2400 Clay Street, San Francisco, CA 94115, USA
* Corresponding author.
E-mail address: drmaas@maasclinic.com

Facial Plast Surg Clin N Am 27 (2019) 419–423
https://doi.org/10.1016/j.fsc.2019.04.009

environment while tempering local tissue reactivity.

DONOR SITES

The importance of donor site selection on grafting predictability remains controversial. Coleman[8] reported no difference in site-specific donor effect on viability based on practice and observation, although no measurements were published. This observation was supported by a study of in vitro adipocyte viability after tissue harvest from four locations in five patients.[9] The long-term results in vivo, however, may be enhanced by increased MSC concentration in the transferred tissue, and the donor sites of the lower abdomen[10] and outer thighs[11] have been shown to produce more of these important cells.

HARVEST

The technique for harvesting roughly follows the direction laid out by Coleman in 1998.[8] A 3- to 5-mm Coleman blunt tip cannula is attached to a 10-mL syringe and advanced through a small stab incision in the skin. With negative pressure held on the syringe, slow controlled passes are made with the cannula deep to the dermis in a fanning pattern to remove tissue evenly from the donor site. Syringes are replaced as they are filled. Powered suction is avoided to reduce tissue trauma and maintain gentle tissue handling from harvest, through preparation, and to injection (**Fig. 1**).

PREPARATION

Centrifugation is the most commonly reported method used for fat preparation, although other

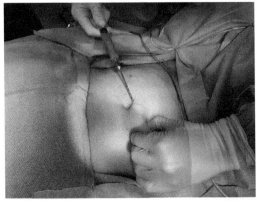

Fig. 1. Fat harvest from the anterior abdomen through a periumbilical stab incision using manual suction with a 10-mL syringe.

methods including decantation, washing through a sieve, and serum absorption with nonadherent sponge are also widely used.[2] Although centrifugation speeds up the process of separating out the harvested components, it also exposes the cells to additional trauma. Centrifugation with high speeds or prolonged force on the fat leads to increased cell death compared with decantation alone.[12,13] Washing through a sieve has been shown to have comparable adipocyte cell viability as high-force, short-duration centrifugation.[13,14] A review of the literature by Gir and colleagues[15] identifies papers touting each of the main preparation techniques as the best for optimal adipocyte viability or quantifiable postoperative results.

With respect to MSCs, washing was shown to have the highest concentration of MSCs within the adipose with decantation procuring fewer MSCs and centrifugation separating MSCs from the fat altogether and lumping them with the cell pellet, which is generally discarded.[16]

Sedimentation is used in our practice. Once the adipose tissue is harvested, filled syringes are placed vertically on the back table with the plunger up and the tip down for a period of about 1 hour to allow nontraumatic separation of the tissue components. Once the components have been allowed time to separate and settle the serum that has accumulated at the tip of the syringe is removed. A funnel-shaped transfer connector is used to connect the 10-mL syringe to a 1-mL syringe. Fat is gently transferred through the funnel connector back and forth between the two syringes until it flows easily. In this way the 1-mL syringes to be used for injection are filled with fat and MSCs (**Fig. 2**).

With the increase in the popularity of fat transfer procedures, novel devices seeking to streamline the process, decrease variability in steps, or preferentially harvest certain tissue components have come and gone from the market. Currently PureGraft (PureGraft, Solana Beach, CA) and Lipogems (Lipogems International S.P.A, Milano, Italy) are among the offerings of patented processing devices. Published reports by those affiliated with the companies report that PureGraft optimally removes contaminant from the fat[17] and Lipogems preferentially harvests MSCs[18,19] (Video 1).

INJECTION TECHNIQUES

Injection of the processed tissue is performed with a needle or blunt tip cannula (Video 2). It is most frequently administered as small aliquots of less than 0.1 mL per pass in a fanning technique.[2,20] Additionally, there is literature to support that harvested fat can be frozen and stored using a

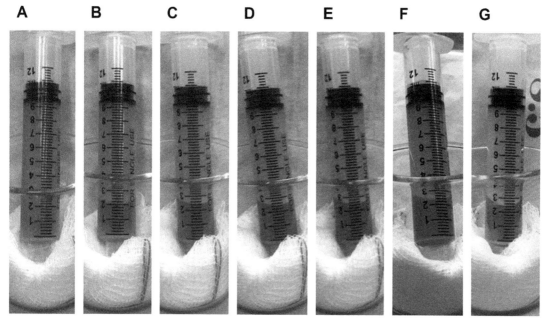

Fig. 2. Time lapse of fat harvested allowing separation by sedimentation. Images show fat at (*A*) 0 minutes, (*B*) 3 minutes, (*C*) 6 minutes, (*D*) 9 minutes, (*E*) 15 minutes, (*F*) 37 minutes, and (*G*) 63 minutes.

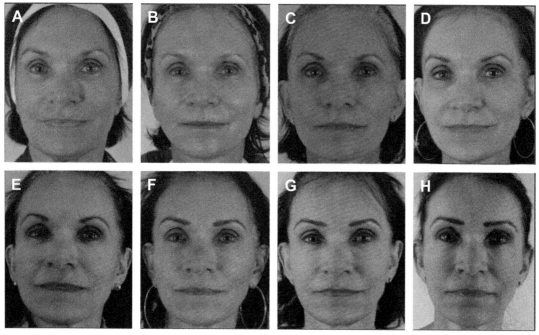

Fig. 3. Patient before and after fat transfer with accompanying lower facelift, submental liposuction, chemical peel, and fractional laser resurfacing. Images show the appearance of the midface progression preoperatively and postoperatively. The patient received 8.5 mL of processed lipoaspirate to the right midface and 5.5 mL to the left midface because of facial volume discrepancy between the sides. Images show preoperative (*A*) and postoperative images at 2 weeks (*B*), 1 month (*C*), 2 months (*D*), 7 months (*E*), 9 months (*F*), 12 months (*G*), and 15 months (*H*) after the procedures.

cryoprecipitate.[15] Overcorrecting is performed by some practitioners because of anticipated fat loss with time, but patients must be counseled regarding the potential appearance of severe over-correction caused by post-procedural edema (**Fig. 3**).[21]

PEARLS

- Tissue harvesting and processing should be gentle to avoid unnecessary adipose destruction.
- The processing technique used should maximize the retention of MSCs for injection to aid in mitigation of the immune response to grafting and creation of a local environment maximizing adipocyte integration and differentiation.
- Donor site selection, processing technique, and portions of the processed tissue used for fat transfer can impact the chance of successful tissue transplantation.

SUPPLEMENTARY DATA

Supplementary data related to this article can be found online at https://doi.org/10.1016/j.fsc.2019.04.009.

REFERENCES

1. Ali MJ, Ende K, Maas CS. Perioral rejuvenation and lip augmentation. Facial Plast Surg Clin North Am 2007;15(4):491–500.
2. Sinno S, Mehta K, Reavey PL, et al. Current trends in facial rejuvenation: an assessment of ASPS members' use of fat grafting during face lifting. Plast Reconstr Surg 2015;136(1):20e–30e. Available at: https://journals.lww.com/plasreconsurg/Fulltext/2015/07000/Current_Trends_in_Facial_Rejuvenation___An.7.aspx.
3. Krastev TK, Beugels J, Hommes J, et al. Efficacy and safety of autologous fat transfer in facial reconstructive surgery: a systematic review and meta-analysis. JAMA Facial Plast Surg 2018;20(5):351–60.
4. Caplan AI. Mesenchymal stem cells: time to change the name! Stem Cells Transl Med 2017;6(6):1445–51.
5. Salinas HM, Broelsch GF, Fernandes JR, et al. Comparative analysis of processing methods in fat grafting. Plast Reconstr Surg 2014;134(4):675–83. Available at: https://journals.lww.com/plasreconsurg/Fulltext/2014/10000/Comparative_Analysis_of_Processing_Methods_in_Fat.17.aspx.
6. da Silva Meirelles L, Fontes AM, Covas DT, et al. Mechanisms involved in the therapeutic properties of mesenchymal stem cells. Cytokine Growth Factor Rev 2009;20(5):419–27.
7. Murphy MB, Moncivais K, Caplan AI. Mesenchymal stem cells: environmentally responsive therapeutics for regenerative medicine. Exp Mol Med 2013;45(11):e54.
8. Coleman SR. Structural fat grafting. Aesthet Surg J 1998;18(5):386–8.
9. Rohrich RJ, Sorokin ES, Brown SA. In search of improved fat transfer viability: a quantitative analysis of the role of centrifugation and harvest site. Plast Reconstr Surg 2004;113(1):391–5. Available at: https://journals.lww.com/plasreconsurg/Fulltext/2004/01000/In_Search_of_Improved_Fat_Transfer_Viability__A.61.aspx.
10. Padoin AV, Braga-Silva J, Martins P, et al. Sources of processed lipoaspirate cells: influence of donor site on cell concentration. Plast Reconstr Surg 2008;122(2):614–48. Available at: https://journals.lww.com/plasreconsurg/Fulltext/2008/08000/Sources_of_Processed_Lipoaspirate_Cells__Influence.36.aspx.
11. Tsekouras A, Mantas D, Tsilimigras DI, et al. Comparison of the viability and yield of adipose-derived stem cells (ASCs) from different donor areas. In Vivo 2017;31(6):1229–34.
12. Hoareau L, Bencharif K, Girard A-C, et al. Effect of centrifugation and washing on adipose graft viability: a new method to improve graft efficiency. J Plast Reconstr Aesthet Surg 2013;66(5):712–9.
13. Rose JGJ, Lucarelli MJ, Lemke BN, et al. Histologic comparison of autologous fat processing methods. Ophthalmic Plast Reconstr Surg 2006;22(3):195–200. Available at: https://journals.lww.com/op-rs/Fulltext/2006/05000/Histologic_Comparison_of_Autologous_Fat_Processing.10.aspx.
14. Asilian A, Siadat AH, Iraji R. Comparison of fat maintenance in the face with centrifuge versus filtered and washed fat. J Res Med Sci 2014;19(6):556–61.
15. Gir P, Brown SA, Oni G, et al. Fat grafting: evidence-based review on autologous fat harvesting, processing, reinjection, and storage. Plast Reconstr Surg 2012;130(1):249–58. Available at: https://journals.lww.com/plasreconsurg/Fulltext/2012/07000/Fat_Grafting___Evidence_Based_Review_on_Autologous.48.aspx.
16. Condé-Green A, Gontijo de Amorim NF, Pitanguy I. Influence of decantation, washing and centrifugation on adipocyte and mesenchymal stem cell content of aspirated adipose tissue: a comparative study. J Plast Reconstr Aesthet Surg 2010;63(8):1375–81.
17. Zhu M, Cohen SR, Hicok KC, et al. Comparison of three different fat graft preparation methods: gravity separation, centrifugation, and simultaneous washing with filtration in a closed system. Plast Reconstr Surg 2013;131(4):873–80. Available at: https://journals.lww.com/plasreconsurg/Fulltext/2013/04000/Comparison_of_Three_Different_Fat_Graft.40.aspx.

18. Tremolada C, Colombo V, Ventura C. Adipose tissue and mesenchymal stem cells: state of the art and Lipogems® technology development. Curr Stem Cell Rep 2016;2(3):304–12.

19. Bianchi F, Maioli M, Leonardi E, et al. A new nonenzymatic method and device to obtain a fat tissue derivative highly enriched in pericyte-like elements by mild mechanical forces from human lipoaspirates. Cell Transplant 2013; 22(11):2063–77.

20. Maas CS. Botulinum neurotoxins and injectable fillers: minimally invasive management of the aging upper face. Facial Plast Surg Clin North Am 2006; 14(3):241–5.

21. Attenello N. Injectable fillers: review of material and properties. Facial Plast Surg 2015;31(1):29–34.

Moving?

Make sure your subscription moves with you!

To notify us of your new address, find your **Clinics Account Number** (located on your mailing label above your name), and contact customer service at:

Email: journalscustomerservice-usa@elsevier.com

800-654-2452 (subscribers in the U.S. & Canada)
314-447-8871 (subscribers outside of the U.S. & Canada)

Fax number: 314-447-8029

Elsevier Health Sciences Division
Subscription Customer Service
3251 Riverport Lane
Maryland Heights, MO 63043

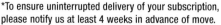
*To ensure uninterrupted delivery of your subscription, please notify us at least 4 weeks in advance of move.

Printed and bound by CPI Group (UK) Ltd, Croydon, CR0 4YY

08/05/2025

01864746-0018